Identifying Filamentous Fungi

A Clinical Laboratory Handbook

Identifying Filamentous Fungi

A Clinical Laboratory Handbook

Guy St-Germain, B.S.
Laboratoire de santé
publique du Québec

Richard Summerbell, Ph.D.
Ontario Ministry of Health

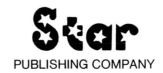

PUBLISHING COMPANY

ISBN 0-89863-177-7 (English edition)

ISBN 0-89863-179-3 (Édition française)

Star Publishing Company
P.O. Box 68
Belmont, California 94002
USA

Printed in Korea
0 9 8 7 6 5 4 3 2 1

Table of contents

Preface

This book is intended to be a practical manual for the laboratory identification of filamentous fungi of medical importance. Currently, in the world of modern medicine, the increasing number of debilitated patients, particularly of immunocompromised patients, has brought about a corresponding increase in the number of serious cases of mycotic disease. These infections are caused by a great variety of opportunistic fungi, of which only some are more-or-less well known. The challenge that their identification represents for the laboratory technologist as well as for the scientist never ceases to grow. In order to alleviate this problem, we present descriptions of 98 genera or species of fungi isolated in the biomedical laboratory. Given that the identification of these organisms rests almost exclusively on morphological examination, we have assigned particular importance to illustrations. Also, to minimize the difficulties occasioned by specialized vocabulary, a glossary is included. We sincerely hope that this guide will facilitate the task of all those who work within this area of medical mycology, while stimulating further interest in those amazing organisms, the filamentous fungi.

Acknowledgements

We thank Lynne Sigler, Edouard Drouhet and Ira Salkin for their most helpful comments and suggestions. We also wish to acknowledge the invaluable assistance of Dominique St-Pierre for photographic expertise, Danielle Beauchesne and Christiane Dion for the preparation of numerous cultures, and Louiselle Clément for illustrations generated by computer. Finally, we wish to thank the many people who have helped us in the preparation and proofreading of our manuscript.

Introduction

Definition

The Kingdom Fungi contains a diversity of organisms, including macroscopic forms as well as filamentous or yeast-like microscopic structures. Fungi are found throughout nature and they play a vital role in the recycling of organic matter. They are often referred to as "saprophytes" or "saprobes", that is, organisms which draw their nourishment from decomposing organic matter. Characteristically, they are eukaryotes, with unicellular or multicellular structures bounded by a rigid cell wall containing chitin. Unlike plants, they do not produce chlorophyll and obtain nourishment only by absorption of carbon from external sources. They are considered phylogenetically distinct from both plants and animals in their unique synthesis of L-lysine by the L-∝-amino-adipic acid pathway. The principal type of sterol present in their cell membranes is ergosterol. Finally, the fungi, in addition to reproducing asexually, often possess a form of sexual reproduction. This is reflected in a very distinctive manner at the level of their classification, as many species bear two names, one designating their asexual state (anamorph) and the other their sexual state (teleomorph) (Kwon-Chung and Bennett 1992, Rippon 1988).

Classification

The organisms featured in this book are arranged in Table 1 according to their divisions, classes, orders and families. Medically important fungi in general belong to the divisions Ascomycota, Basidiomycota or Zygomycota, in accordance with the tendency of sexually reproducing forms to produce ascospores, basidiospores, or zygospores (Fig. 1). Certain species are homothallic and are able to form sexual structures automatically within a single colony. The majority, however, are heterothallic and form their sexual structures only upon the crossing of two compatible strains of differing mating type. Sexual reproduction is often difficult to obtain in the laboratory. This fact largely explains the great number of fungi that were first described exclusively in their asexual form, and were placed in the division Fungi Imperfecti (Deuteromycota). For example, *Microsporum canis* was initially classified in the class Hyphomycetes of the division

1

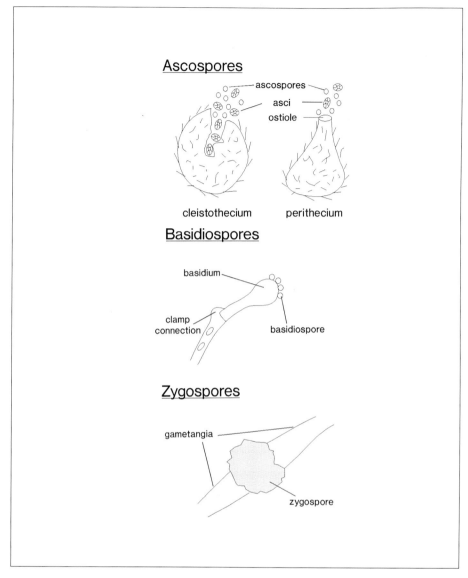

Figure 1.   Sexually reproducing forms belonging to the divisions
             Ascomycota, Basidiomycota or Zygomycota, in
             accordance with the production of ascospores,
             basidiospores, or zygospores .

Fungi Imperfecti based on its asexually produced macroconidia. Later, after this dermatophyte was shown to be able
to reproduce sexually by the formation of ascospores, it was
also integrated into the division Ascomycota where it now
bears the name *Arthroderma otae*. Once a teleomorph is
known, certain mycologists advocate that the name of the
asexual state no longer be used. In practice, however, the
anamorph name often remains the most important and most
widely used. It must be noted also that numerous species

classified in the Fungi Imperfecti have not, as yet, ever been observed to form a sexual state, and thus possess only a single name.

Criteria of identification

The identification of filamentous fungi depends mainly on the morphological examination of microscopic structures, particularly the spores and the conidia, as well as the specialized cells which produce them. An organism which does not sporulate will often be impossible to identify; therefore, it is important to choose culture conditions which favour sporulation. In addition, even though subject to a degree of variability, the appearance and growth rate of colonies are useful identification features.

Colony appearance

The texture and colour of colonies can be influenced by the culture medium used or by the age of the isolate, but nonetheless remain typical of genera or of species. Whereas some colonies have a glabrous appearance because they form few aerial hyphae, others are woolly or powdery. Some colonies are pale in colour (whitish, beige, yellowish, pinkish) while others are brightly coloured (green, yellow, cinnamon, pink, red, mauve, violet). Fungi referred to as "dematiaceous" (family Dematiaceae, class Hyphomycetes) possess a brown, melanin-type pigment in their cell walls; this explains the dull colours (grey, brown, olive-brown, black) of their colonies. In some, the pigment is concentrated in their conidia, so that their colonies appear dark on the surface and pale or colourless on the reverse. Those which elaborate melanin within the hyphal walls possess colonies which are darkened on both the surface and the reverse.

Growth rate

The culture medium, the incubation temperature, and the amount of inoculum used are all factors which influence the colony growth rate. Nonetheless, under controlled conditions, the growth rate remains sufficiently constant that it can be taken into consideration in the process of identification. For example, certain dermatophytes develop very slowly, their colonies not exceeding 0.5 cm in diameter after 1 week of incubation; in comparison, certain Mucorales such as *Rhizopus* cover the entire surface of a 9 cm petri plate in as little as 2 to 3 days.

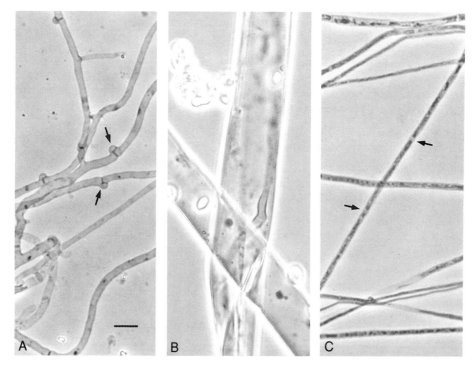

Figure 2.   Different types of hyphae: A) hyphae with clamp connections↑ of *Schizophyllum commune*, B) large, aseptate or few-septate hyphae of *Rhizopus* sp., C) narrow, septate↑ hyphae of *Trichophyton rubrum*.

Hyphae

Three major categories of hyphae (Fig. 2) may aid in the recognition of certain groups of fungi: 1) large, aseptate or few-septate hyphae are characteristic of the Zygomycetes and more specifically the Mucorales (*Rhizopus, Mucor, Absidia*, etc.); 2) vegetative hyphae with clamp connections indicate a fungus in the division Basidiomycota, but these hyphae are rarely seen in the biomedical laboratory; and 3) relatively narrow, septate hyphae are characteristic of the great majority of medically important filamentous fungi.

Sexual reproduction

For all practical purposes, in the clinical laboratory, filamentous fungi which spontaneously produce their sexually reproductive structures (that is, homothallic fungi) are few and are limited in routine observation to a few species, namely *Aspergillus nidulans, Aspergillus glaucus* gr., *Chaetomium*, and *Pseudallescheria boydii*. These organisms produce fruiting bodies called "ascomata" (in older literature "ascocarps") which are often observed as spherical or flask-shaped structures containing asci at first, then, at maturity, free ascospores. Two types are readily encountered (Fig. 1): the perithecium, which disperses its spores by extruding or shooting them through an apical opening called an ostiole, and the cleistothecium, which, lacking a specialized opening, splits under pressure and thus liberates its contents.

Asexual reproduction

The overwhelming majority of medically important filamentous fungi are identified by the morphology of their specialized asexual structures (conidia, asexual spores or conidiogenous cells) which are key, even indispensable, elements used in the recognition of genera and species. The most common zygomycete genera, for example, are distinguished from one another by the morphology of their sporangiophores, sporangia, and sporangiospores, as well as by the presence or absence of rhizoids. In the Hyphomycetes, a class containing the great majority of medically important filamentous fungi, the conidia are often categorized into those formed through a blastic process or through a thallic process. Blastic conidia are produced in a process that is in essence an act of budding; there is considerable or substantial new wall building in the process of conidial development and the wall separating the new cell from the mother cell appears only at the time of maturation. By contrast, conidia of thallic ontogeny are the product of hyphal segments which are already delimited by a septum. These segments then differentiate as specialized conidia. In practice, given the morphological variability of the numerous species involved, the application of the distinction between blastic and thallic is difficult in a few groups and has been the subject of some controversy (Sigler, 1989, Cole and Samson, 1983). In order to simplify the characterization of conidia commonly seen in the clinical laboratory, we have chosen to classify them into 7 types, the first four produced by a blastic process (Fig. 3), and the remaining 3 produced in a process which is either clearly thallic or at least has a predominantly thallic nature.

Blastoconidia. We consider blastoconidia to be those conidia formed by a budding process at the apex of a conidiophore, or from another conidium. They may be solitary (*Nigrospora, Arthrinium*), or in branched chains (*Cladosporium*); certain types are formed sympodially, on denticles (*Beauveria, Sporothrix*) or through pores (*Alternaria, Bipolaris*), developing in succes-

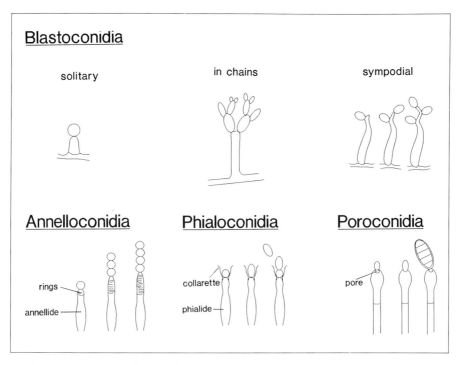

Figure 3. Blastic conidia.

sion as the conidiophore apex extends and tending to form a zigzag or rosette pattern beneath the extending tip.

Phialoconidia. Phialides are typically bottle shaped conidiogenous cells which at their apices produce conidia collecting in mucoid masses (*Fusarium, Acremonium*) or remaining attached to each other in unbranched, dry chains (*Aspergillus, Penicillium*). Their elongation ceases with the production of the initial conidium. In some species, the apices of the phialides are conspicuously adorned with a tubular or cup-shaped membrane referred to as a collarette; the shape of the collarette is a particularly important criterion for identifying species in the genus *Phialophora*.

Annelloconidia. Annellides, like phialides, produce conidia in mucoid masses (*Exophiala, Scedosporium*) or in unbranched chains (*Scopulariopsis*). They are distinguished from phialides by continuing to grow in length during the process of conidiation and by the presence of a series of annular rings at their apex. It should be noted that these rings, which are in fact the scars left behind by successive conidia as they break away from the apex, are often difficult to see under the conventional light microscope. In ordinary practice, when it becomes important to distinguish annellides

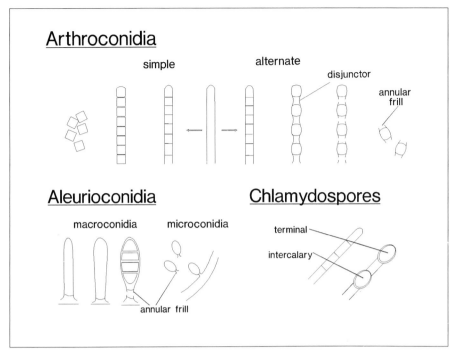

Figure 4.   Thallic conidia, aleurioconidia and resting cells.

from phialides, one must closely examine the extreme apex of the conidiogenous cell. In particular for the identification of certain dematiaceous fungi such as *Phialophora* and *Exophiala*, the annellide tends to be more sharply pointed whereas the phialide appears truncated.

Poroconidia.   Poroconidia are produced through pores in the cell wall of the conidiophore. Besides often being darkly melanized and multiseptate, they are also often produced in a sympodial succession, as is reflected in the geniculate shape of their conidiophores.

Arthroconidia.   Arthroconidia are conidia of thallic origin which arise from the transformation of a series of cells along the length of a hypha. They may be contiguous (simple) or intercalated with separating cells (alternate). At maturity, simple arthroconidia are liberated after the formation of double walls followed by a process of fission, while alternate arthroconidia are liberated after the lysis of the separating cells. In the latter case, annular frills of remnant wall material can be observed at the ends of the detached conidia.

Table I — Classification of Fungi

Kingdom: Fungi

Division: Zygomycota
  Classe: Zygomycetes

Mucorales	*Absidia, Cunninghamella, Mucor, Rhizomucor, Rhizopus, Syncephalastrum*
Entomophthorales	*Basidiobolus, Conidiobolus*

Division: Ascomycota
  Classe: Ascomycetes

Onygenales	*Arthroderma = * Microsporum, Trichophyton, Chrysosporium (in part)* *Ajellomyces = Blastomyces, Histoplasma*
Eurotiales	*Emericella nidulans = Aspergillus nidulans, Eurotium = Aspergillus glaucus gr.* *Pseudallescheria boydii = Scedosporium apiospermum*
Sphaeriales	*Chaetomium, Neurospora = Chrysonilia*

Division: Basidiomycota	*Schizophyllum commune*

Division: Fungi imperfecti (Deuteromycota)
  Classe: Hyphomycetes
    Moniliales

Moniliaceae	*Acremonium, Arthrographis, Aspergillus, Beauveria, Blastomyces, Chrysonilia, Chrysosporium, Coccidioides, Emmonsia, Epidermophyton, Fusarium, Geotrichum, Gliocladium, Histoplasma, Lecythophora, Microsporum, Paecilomyces, Penicillium, Paracoccidioides, Scopulariopsis, Scytalidium, Sepedonium, Sporothrix, Sporotrichum, Stachybotrys, Trichophyton, Trichoderma, Trichothecium, Tritirachium, Verticillium*
Dematiaceae	*Alternaria, Arthrinium, Aureobasidium, Bipolaris, Botrytis, Cladosporium, Curvularia, Dreschlera, Epicoccum, Exserohilum, Exophiala, Fonsecaea, Helminthosporium, Lecythophora, Madurella, Nigrospora, Phialophora, Pithomyces, Rhinocladiella, Scedosporium, Scolecobasidium, Scopulariopsis, Scytalidium, Sporothrix, Stachybotrys, Ulocladium, Wangiella, Xylohypha*
Classe: Coelomycetes	
	Phoma, Nattrassia

*"=" indicates an anamorph teleomorph relationship.

Chlamydospores. Traditionally the term chlamydospore has been used for environmentally resistant resting cells which, somewhat like arthroconidia, are formed from pre-existing cells within a hypha. These are the inflated, more or less rounded cells with thick walls frequently present in older cultures. In contrast to spores and conidia, they lack a dehiscence mechanism allowing them to detach from the fungal thallus when mature. Although generally too nonspecific to be useful in diagnosis, they can sometimes serve as an identification marker for certain species, such as the dermatophyte *Trichophyton verrucosum*.

Aleurioconidia. Aleurioconidia are terminally or laterally formed conidia liberated by the lysis of the cells which support them. They are usually recognized by their truncate bases bearing small annular frills, these frills being remnants of the walls of supporting cells which lysed during the process of dehiscence. This type of conidium is characteristic of the dermatophytes and several other fungi of medical or clinical laboratory interest such as *Chrysosporium*, *Histoplasma*, and *Blastomyces*. Some aleurioconidia are formed by a process which in some ways appears typically thallic; yet, at the same time, many tend to inflate peripherally during formation in a way that resembles blastic conidiation. This has led to their being referred to as blastoconidia in some literature.

Laboratory safety

Several organizations have published guidelines for laboratory safety in microbiology (Centers for Disease Control and National Institutes of Health, 1988, Medical Research Council of Canada, 1990, World Health Organization, 1993). The specific recommendations may sometimes vary but essentially, they concur that the great majority of fungi present little hazard to the healthy individual. Only the dimorphic fungi *Coccidioides immitis*, *Blastomyces dermatitidis*, *Histoplasma capsulatum*, and *Paracoccidioides brasiliensis* are considered dangerous in their sporulating phase, presenting a high degree of risk to individuals exposed to them. Sporulating cultures of these organisms should therefore never be opened except in a type I or type II biological safety cabinet, in a containment laboratory.

The inhalation of infectious conidia of the dimorphic fungi is the origin of most of the mycoses acquired in the biomedical laboratory. As a general rule, when examining any sporulating culture, the laboratorian should pay special attention to any manipulations which may allow conidia to escape into the air. It suffices to recall that these particles constitute the principal means of dissemination of fungi in nature, and they may be carried by the least current of air. Also, the careless manipulation of sporulating cultures, besides sometimes presenting a risk of infection or allergy, may also bring about the contamination of laboratory air and create difficulties in other activities, such as, for example, the contamination of bacterial cultures.

As a general rule, it is recommended that all bodily specimens (respiratory secretions, biopsies, and others) which may contain dangerous infectious agents transmissible by aerosolization (mycobacteria, viruses) be manipulated in a biological safety cabinet. This practice also diminishes the risk of infection by dimorphic fungal pathogens. Even though these fungi present a lesser risk in the context of primary isolation, sporulating cultures should be manipulated in a biological safety cabinet in a containment laboratory. The sporulating cultures of other filamentous fungi such as dermatophytes and the saprophytes in general may be manipulated on the laboratory bench outside the safety cabinet; however, it is standard practice today to have safety cabinets suitable for work with fungi installed during the construction or renovation of the laboratory.

Identification

Two identification keys are given here, one dichotomous and the other illustrated. The first requires knowledge of terminology used in mycology (see Glossary for assistance) while the second depends primarily on the comparison of microscopic structures.

Before beginning, the user of these keys should understand that neither key permits the identification of all the genera or species which may be isolated in the biomedical laboratory. Many of the more rare organisms are not included. Some species which occur in numerous variant forms are treated here only in their most typical form. Thus, once a name for an unknown isolate has been found, using the criteria or illustrations given, the accuracy of the identification should be confirmed by ascertaining that the major characters of the genus or species being considered are truly compatible with the unknown isolate. These characters are detailed in the technical descriptions in this book or in other specialized literature, and should be referred to each time a new identification is made. Where there is doubt, the judgement of a reference laboratory should be solicited.

Dichotomous key to the genera and species treated

1. Hyphae aseptate or few-septate, often > 4 μm in diameter; sporangia, merosporangia or sporangioles present; ballistospores or zygospores occasionally present. 2

1a. Hyphae septate, variable in diameter but often < 4 μm; dematiaceous or hyaline yeasts sometimes present or even predominant in the early stages of colony growth 9

Zygomycetes

2. Ballistospores (ejectable sporangioles) present; zygospores sometimes present. 3

2a. Ballistospores and zygospores absent 4

3. Sporangiophores inflated apically; ejected ballistospores retaining a fragment of the sporangiophore at the base; beaked zygospores frequently present. . . . . *Basidiobolus*

3a. Sporangiophores not or scarcely inflated; ejected ballistospores show a papilla but no sporangiophore remnant at the base; zygospores lacking beaks sometimes present. . . . . *Conidiobolus*

4. Spores formed in masses within sporangia 5

4a. Spores formed within sporangioles or merosporangia attached to the surface of a rounded vesicle 8

5. Sporangia round; sporangiophores solitary or in clusters, with well developed rhizoids at the base . . . . *Rhizopus*

5a. Sporangia pear-shaped, broadly oval or sometimes round; rhizoids absent, rudimentary or produced at sites other than the base of the sporangiophores
. . . . 6

6.   Funnel-shaped apophysis present beneath the
        sporangium; rhizoids present. . . . . *Absidia*

6a.   Apophysis absent; rhizoids absent or rudimentary
        7

7.   Growth at 54°C; rudimentary rhizoids present but
        often difficult to recognize . . . . *Rhizomucor*

7a.   No growth at 54°C; rhizoids absent . . . . *Mucor*

8.   (from 4a) Spores formed individually within
        sporangioles attached to individual denticles on
        the surface of a round vesicle. . . . . *Cunninghamella*

8a.   Spores formed in linear series within
        merosporangia attached to the surface of a round
        vesicle. . . . . *Syncephalastrum*

---

9.   (from 1a) Complex reproductive structures
        present, either sexual (cleistothecia, perithecia) or
        asexual (pycnidia). 10

9a.   Complex reproductive structures absent 13

**Fungi producing complex reproductive
structures, either sexual (cleistothecia or
perithecia - Ascomycetes) or asexual
(pycnidia - Coelomycetes)**

10.   Complex reproductive structures (perithecia)
        greyish olive green to black, covered with long,
        sinuous, spiralling or erect setae; ascospores dark
        brown, often lemon- shaped. . . . . *Chaetomium*

10a.   Reproductive structures glabrous or covered with
        short bristles 11

11.   *Scedosporium*-type oval conidia with truncate
        bases present; complex reproductive structures
        (cleistothecia) glabrous; ascospores ellipsoidal,
        orange-brown . . . . *Pseudallescheria boydii*

11a. *Scedosporium*-type conidia absent 12

12. Complex reproductive structures (cleistothecia) glabrous, accompanied by *Aspergillus* heads; colony green or yellow. 114

12a. Complex reproductive structures (pycnidia) glabrous or covered with short bristles, ostiolate, producing large quantities of viscous, usually pale conidia; colony often pinkish grey . . . . *Phoma*

13. Colony dark (pigmented grey, olive brown, brown or black); in some cases the colony is pale in early growth and becomes darkened in age 14

13a. Colony pale or brightly coloured (yellow, green, golden, cinnamon, red, violet). 53

14. Colony failing to produce conidia after 14 days. 15

14a. Colony producing conidia. 17

Sterile dark fungi

15. Fungus isolated from a mycetoma and associated with the presence of black granules; colonies brownish to grey and often producing a brown soluble pigment 16

15a. Other nonsporulating cultures; attempt to induce production of conidia by using a medium favouring sporulation, such as potato glucose agar or 2% water agar. If the isolate remains sterile and fails to grow at 37°C . . . . sterile dark contaminant

16. Good growth at 37°C; sucrose assimilated . . . . *Madurella mycetomatis*

14

16a.   Growth at 37°C weak or absent; sucrose not assimilated. . . . . *Madurella grisea*

17.   Colony slimy or pasty in texture, producing budding yeast cells in great or small quantity, at least in early growth; hyphae in some cases not appearing until after 2 to 3 weeks of incubation. 18

17a.   Colony typically cottony or woolly; yeast cells absent 22

Dematiaceous fungi producing yeast cells

18.   Colony initially whitish, pale rose, pale yellow, or pale brown, becoming dark brown to black with the appearance of brown hyphae which may break down to form arthroconidia or chlamydospores . . . . *Aureobasidium*

18a.   Colony dark even in initial phases of growth. . . 19

19.   Yeast cells often bicellular, with a roughened end giving rise to annelloconidia . . . . *Exophiala werneckii*

19a.   Yeast cells strictly unicellular 20

20.   Unicellular conidia produced on phialides lacking collarettes; growth occurs at 40°C; potassium nitrate not assimilated. . . . . . *Wangiella dermatitidis*

20a.   Unicellular conidia produced on annellides; no growth at 40°C; potassium nitrate assimilated . . 21

21.   Conidia produced on cylindrical or somewhat inflated annellides; conidiophore often consists of a single cell or is absent altogether . . . . *Exophiala jeanselmei*

21a.   Conidia produced on spine-like annellides, often
        supported by a conidiophore consisting of 2 to 4
        cells . . . . *Exophiala spinifera*

22.   (from 17a) Conidia mostly multicellular
        (more than 2 cells). 23

22a.   Conidia unicellular and/or bicellular. 31

**Dematiaceous fungi producing
multicellular conidia**

---

23.   Muriform conidia present - that is, conidia with
        septa both in the longitudinal and transverse
        planes. 24

23a.   Conidia with transverse septa only 27

24.   Conidia (aleurioconidia) with wide, truncate
        bases, produced on short conidiophores little
        differentiated from vegetative hyphae; a fragment
        of the conidiophore wall (annular frill) remains
        attached to the base of the detached conidia. . . . 25

24a.   Conidia (poroconidia) often produced on a
        geniculate conidiophore; annular frill absent from
        the base of detached conidia 26

25.   Conidia mostly ellipsoidal; colony pale becoming
        brown to grey . . . . *Pithomyces*

25a.   Conidia rather round, with warty exterior; colony
        yellow to red, becoming rusty brown to black
        . . . . *Epicoccum*

26.   Conidia obclavate with beak-shaped apical cell,
        often in chains; conidiogenous cell not or only
        slightly geniculate at the apex . . . . *Alternaria*

26a.   Conidia ovoid to ellipsoidal, without a beak-like
        extension at the extremity, most commonly
        solitary, rarely in short chains; conidiogenous
        cell usually strongly geniculate at the apex
        . . . . *Ulocladium*

27.   Conidia obclavate, produced along the sides of a
        long, erect conidiophore with determinate growth
        . . . . *Helminthosporium*

27a.   Conidia ellipsoidal, cylindrical, or curved, formed
        sympodially on a geniculate conidiophore 28

28.   Conidia often curved; central cell asymmetrical,
        larger and darker than the other cells . . *Curvularia*

28a.   Conidia straight or, if curved, without a
        prominently larger and darker central cell 29

29.   Conidia with a protuberant basal scar (hilum)
        . . . . *Exserohilum*

29a.   Conidia lacking a protuberant hilum 30

30.   Germ tubes formed along the longitudinal axis of
        the conidia, emerging from terminal cells
        . . . . *Bipolaris*

30a.   Germ tubes formed perpendicularly to the
        longitudinal axis of the conidia, emerging from
        any cell. . . . . *Drechslera*

Dematiaceous fungi producing unicellular or bicellular conidia

31.   (from 22a) Conidia in chains produced at the
        apex of conidiogenous cells (blastoconidia,
        phialoconidia or annelloconidia) or produced by
        the fragmentation of hyphae (arthroconidia) . . . 32

31a.   Conidia solitary or in sticky masses 39

32.   Brown arthroconidia present. 33

32a.   Arthroconidia absent. 34

33.   Colonies woolly, yeast phase absent . . . *Scytalidium*

33a.   Colony slimy or pasty; yeasts present
        . . . . *Aureobasidium*

34. Conidia in branched chains 35

34a. Conidia in unbranched chains. 38

35. Conidia produced in strongly branched chains containing successive ranks of progressively smaller cells; each of the largest conidia at the base of conidial chains gives rise to 2 - 5 smaller conidia which, at maturity, will form another rank of still smaller conidia; in addition, conidiogenous structures of the *Cladosporium* and *Rhinocladiella* types often present . . . . . . *Fonsecaea*

35a. Conidia in infrequently branched chains; most conidia give rise only to a single daughter conidium, sometimes to two (thereby creating a branch point) and rarely to three. 36

36. Chains of conidia rarely branching at more than one location, resistant to disarticulation, often containing 30 or more conidia; growth at 42°C . . . . *Xylohypha bantiana*

36a. Conidial chains usually branching at more than one location and breaking apart more readily; no growth at 42°C. 37

37. Conidia unicellular; colonies slow growing, black, capable of growth at 35°C . . . . *Cladosporium carrionii*

37a. Conidia mostly unicellular, the larger ones sometimes bicellular (rarely multicellular) and shield shaped; colonies greenish grey to black, moderately rapidly growing, often incapable of growing at 35°C . . . . *Cladosporium*
(species considered normally nonpathogenic)

38. (from 34a) Conidia round, with strongly roughened wall, produced in chains from aspergilloid heads consisting of biseriate phialides attached to the surface of a vesicle, this vesicle situated at the apex of a thick-walled conidiophore . . . . *Aspergillus niger*

38a. Conidia ellipsoidal or lemon shaped, with truncate base, produced in chains from short and basally inflated annellides; annellides often solitary or occasionally clustered
.... *Scopulariopsis brumptii*

39. (from 31a) Colony rapidly growing, white, cottony to velvety; giving rise to black spots on the surface when conidia form after 7- 10 days incubation; mature conidia dark brown with germ slit 40

39a. Colony not as above; conidia without germ slits 41

40. Conidia brown and lens-shaped, measuring less than 12 µm, produced in dry clumps
.... *Arthrinium*

40a. Conidia black, ellipsoidal, dorsiventrally flattened, measuring more than 12 µm across, solitary
.... *Nigrospora*

41. Conidia produced individually on short denticles formed at the apex of the conidiophore 42

41a. Conidia produced on phialides or annellides... 45

42. Conidia mostly bicellular .... *Scolecobasidium*

42a. Conidia unicellular 43

43. Conidiophore broader than the vegetative hyphae, with an apex composed of vesicles covered with denticles, each denticle supporting a single conidium .... *Botrytis*

43a. Conidiophores approximately the same diameter as vegetative hyphae 44

44.   Primary conidia hyaline, obovoid, clustered in rosettes around the apex of the conidiophore; brown secondary conidia formed along the sides of hyphae; colony often glabrous; filamentous colonial form converts to a hyaline yeast form at 37°C on brain-heart infusion agar
.... *Sporothrix schenckii*

44a.   Conidia arranged on denticles all along the sides of the conidiophore apex; colony cottony; black yeast cells sometimes present ..... *Rhinocladiella*

45.   (from 41a) Conidia often solitary, with narrow truncate base, arising from annellides (these conidiogenous cells frequently resemble a narrowly cylindrical hypha with a narrowly truncate tip; occasionally, a series of obscurely bulging annular rings can be seen near the apex) 46

45a.   Conidia produced in sticky masses from phialides (in contrast to the annellide, the phialide often has a readily visible collarette at the apex) 47

46.   Annellides scarcely differentiated from vegetative hyphae; *Pseudallescheria* cleistothecia sometimes present at maturity
.... *Scedosporium apiospermum*

46a.   Annellides with a strongly inflated base; cleistothecia absent ..... *Scedosporium prolificans*

47.   Phisalides with readily visible collarettes 48

47a.   Phialides or adelophialides lacking evident collarettes............................... 51

48.   Phialides flask-shaped, with a conspicuous vase- or saucer- shaped collarette 49

48a.   Phialides cylindrical with a tubular collarette (sometimes inconspicuous)............... 50

49.   Collarettes vase-shaped; conidia cylindrical, hyaline, slightly curved .... *Phialophora verrucosa*

20

49a. Two types of collarette present in mature colonies: phialides with vase-shaped collarettes produce hyaline, cylindrical, slightly curved conidia, while phialides with saucer-shaped collarettes produce round, pale brown conidia
      . . . . *Phialophora richardsiae*

50.   Phialides long, narrowly spiny in shape; conidia cylindrical, slightly curved, colony pale at first becoming grey brown; hyphae with warty walls often present . . . . *Phialophora parasitica*

50a. Phialides rather short, sometimes sinuous, with small, tubular collarettes or sometimes lacking visible collarettes; colony red brown to medium brown; hyphae with warty walls lacking
      . . . . *Phialophora repens*

51.   (from 47a) Colony with a viscous or yeast-like appearance, pink to salmon becoming dark brown; adelophialides predominant; dark brown chlamydospores present at maturity
      . . . . *Lecythophora mutabilis*

51a. Colony cottony to woolly; most phialides are delimited by basal septa 52

52.   Phialides long and narrow, solitary, producing large numbers of slimy, greenish black conidia which, as they accumulate, bring about a colour change of the colony as a whole
      . . . .*Acremonium (Gliomastix)*

52a. Phialides cylindrical, in compact clusters of 4 - 5 at the apex of the conidiophore; conidia black, cylindrical, with smooth or rough surface
      . . . . *Stachybotrys*

53.   (from 13a) Colony not producing conidia after 14 days of growth. 54

53a. Colony producing conidia 64

54.   Growth at 48°C; white mold isolated from
        respiratory tract; growth on medium with
        cycloheximide (e.g. Mycosel) somewhat restricted
        compared to cycloheximide-free control
        . . . . *Aspergillus fumigatus* (sterile)

54a.   No growth at 48°C. 55

55.   Colony growing at 37°C and resistant to
        cycloheximide (growth on Mycosel agar
        incubated at 25°C.) 56

55a.   Colony not growing at 37°C or susceptible to
        cycloheximide . . . . sterile contaminant

56.   Colony isolated from dry dermatologic specimen
        (skin scales, hair, nails) 57

56a.   Colony isolated from deep or subcutaneous
        sites; if a dimorphic fungus is suspected (e.g.,
        *Coccidioides, Blastomyces, Histoplasma,
        Paracoccidioides*), perform tests appropriate to the
        organism(s) suspected, such as examination for
        conversion to a yeast phase at 37°C on rich media
        or exoantigen or probe tests 88, 89, 90, 102

Normally sterile dermatophytes

57.   Colony glabrous to waxy, very slow growing
        (diameter often less than 0.5 cm after 7 days
        growth at 25°C.) 58

57a.   Colony cottony or velvety, with growth slow to
        moderately rapid (diameter over 0.5 cm at 7 days)
        63

58.   Growth dependent on, or strongly stimulated by,
        one or more growth substances as evidenced on
        Trichophyton agars. 59

58a.   No stimulation by growth substances 60

59.   Colony red purple; growth stimulated by thiamine
        . . . . *Trichophyton violaceum*

59a.   Colony white, greyish or yellowish; growth
        stimulated by thiamine and often also by inositol;
        chains of chlamydospores typically present
        . . . . *Trichophyton verrucosum*

60.   Colony rusty to white, pale yellow on
        Lowenstein-Jensen medium; bamboo hyphae
        present . . . . *Microsporum ferrugineum*

60a.   Colony not as above 61

61.   Colony cream-coloured, glabrous, heaped, slowly
        becoming chocolate brown in age, with a brown
        diffusing pigment discolouring the agar
        . . . . *Trichophyton yaoundei*

61a.   Colony not as above 62

62.   Isolate clinically associated with favus; colony
        whitish, heaped; hyphae with tips swollen into
        "nail head" forms or favic chandeliers present
        . . . . *Trichophyton schoenleinii*

62a.   Isolate producing a dermatophytosis of the
        glabrous skin characterised by the formation of
        concentric rings of shingle-like scales; colony
        cerebriform, white to orange brown; isolated only
        from indigenous populations in Indonesia,
        Polynesia, Melanesia, southeast Asia, and central
        America . . . . *Trichophyton concentricum*

63.   (from 57a) Colony low velvety, sulfur yellow to
        apricot or rusty orange, with a peripheral fringe of
        radiating hyphae; reverse brown to red brown;
        deep brown to blackish pigment on
        Lowenstein-Jensen medium; reflexive branches
        present . . . . *Trichophyton soudanense*

63a.   Colony downy, greyish; reverse pale salmon, most
        notably on potato glucose agar; little or no growth
        on polished rice medium but brownish pigment
        discolouring rice . . . . *Microsporum audouinii*

23

Dermatophytes and other sporulating fungi isolated from skin, hair and nails

67.   Unicellular microconidia with rough or smooth walls present; macroconidia absent (a few species produce a small proportion of 2-celled conidia); conidia sometimes formed as short chains of 2-3 cells separated by short hyphal segments; conidiophores sometimes in a tree-like arrangement with side branches diverging at a 45° angle from the principal branch; arthroconidia often present . . . . *Chrysosporium*

67a. Unicellular microconidia, if present, smooth walled; conidia never formed as short terminal chains; multicellular macroconidia, if present, with wall rough or smooth; conidiophores always branching at 90° where branches present; arthroconidia usually absent (but may be present in some isolates of *Trichophyton rubrum* and *T. mentagrophytes* - see key couplet 85) 68

68. Macroconidia fusoid, composed of 3 or more cells, or ovoid, principally 2 - celled 69

68a. Macroconidia absent or, if present, club-shaped or cylindrical 74

69. Macroconidia bicellular, ovoid
. . . . *Microsporum nanum*

69a. Macroconidia multicellular, fusoid 70

70. Macroconidia asymmetrical, with a markedly thick, roughened cell wall. 71

70a. Macroconidia symmetrical, with wall thin or thick, smooth or roughened 72

71. Colony white to yellow with reverse deep yellow to orange; macroconidia with slightly curving apical beak. . . . . *Microsporum canis*

71a. Colony off-white with pale salmon reverse; macroconidia rare, deformed
. . . . *Microsporum audouinii*

72. Microconidia numerous and often on pedicels
. . . . *Microsporum persicolor*

72a. Microconidia few or absent, rarely on pedicels 73

73. Macroconidia with thin, rough walls; colony powdery, beige to cinnamon with reverse yellowish to brown; microconidia present but often few in number . . . . *Microsporum gypseum*

73a. Macroconidia with thick, smooth walls; colony cottony, orange-brown on the surface and often pigmented blue-black on the reverse; microconidia absent or rare . . . *Trichophyton ajelloi*

74. (from 68a) Microconidia absent; the only aleurioconidia formed are thin-walled, club-shaped macroconidia, often produced in clusters; colony olive brown to yellow; growth slow . . . . *Epidermophyton floccosum*

74a. Microconidia more or less numerous, but present; macroconidia often absent. 75

75. Colony glabrous, white or red purple, with very slow growth (small colonies with diameter < 0.5 cm at 7 days) 76

75a. Colony cottony, velvety or powdery, with growth rapid or slow; surface white, beige, yellowish, rusty, reddish or pinkish 77

76. Colony whitish on surface and reverse; chains of chlamydospores typically present from the beginning of colony growth; growth stimulated by thiamin and often also by inositol . . . . *Trichophyton verrucosum*

76a. Colony red purple on the surface and the reverse; chlamydospores present especially in older colonies; growth stimulated only by thiamin . . . . *Trichophyton violaceum*

77. Colony white to pinkish with a red soluble pigment diffusing into the agar (this pigment often produces a red halo measuring twice the diameter of the colony) . . . . . *Microsporum gallinae*

77a. Red pigment absent or, if present, integral to the colony and diffusing little or not at all within the agar. 78

78. Growth weak or absent at 37°C compared to 25°C 79

78a.   Rate of growth similar or faster at 37°C compared
       to 25°C 80

79.   Colony creamy or peach-pink with reverse
       red-brown or pinkish; growth at 37°C weak;
       microconidia pyriform, often on pedicels,
       numerous; clavate to fusoid macroconidia
       sometimes present. . . . . *Microsporum persicolor*

79a.   Colony white with reverse yellowish or sometimes
       red; no growth at 37°C; microconidia club-shaped,
       long, sometimes septate, numerous; 2-4 celled
       cylindrical macroconidia usually present
       . . . . *Trichophyton terrestre*

80.   Colony slow growing, white, yellow, rusty, or
       brown; growth stimulated by thiamin or,
       alternatively, not well supported by any of the
       Trichophyton agars. 81

80a.   Colony with slow to moderately rapid growth,
       white, yellowish, pinkish or reddish; the growth of
       certain species is stimulated by histidine or
       nicotinic acid in the *Trichophyton* agar series . . . 82

81.   Colony low velvety, sulfur yellow to apricot or
       rusty orange, with a peripheral fringe of radiating
       hyphae; microconidia rare; growth slow or absent
       on *Trichophyton* agars, with no evidence of specific
       dependence; reflexive branches typically present
       . . . . *Trichophyton soudanense*

81a.   Colony powdery to velvety, white, beige, yellow or
       brown with reverse yellowish or red-brown;
       numerous microconidia of various forms and sizes
       present (pyriform, club-shaped, balloon forms);
       growth stimulated by thiamin; reflexive branches
       absent. . . . . *Trichophyton tonsurans*

82.   Growth stimulated by histidine or nicotinic
       acid 83

82a.   No special nutritional requirements. 84

83.   Colony yellowish; growth rapid, stimulated
        by nicotinic acid
        . . . . *Trichophyton equinum* var. *equinum*

83a.   Colony pinkish or reddish; growth moderately
        rapid, stimulated by histidine
        . . . . *Trichophyton megninii*

84.   Colony off-white to greyish; pale salmon pigment
        present in the reverse particularly on potato
        glucose agar; poor growth on polished rice
        medium; microconidia often rare; macroconidia
        rare, deformed . . . . *Microsporum audouinii*

84a.   Colony white, pinkish or reddish; reverse pale,
        yellowish, brown or red; microconidia sometimes
        abundant 85

85.   Colony cottony to powdery, white to pinkish,
        typically with blood red pigment on the reverse
        (isolates which fail to produce red pigment on
        Sabouraud agar will usually do so on potato
        glucose agar); pencil shaped macroconidia
        sometimes present; urease and *in vitro* hair
        perforation tests negative; no change of pH on
        BCP milk solids glucose agar at 7 days of
        incubation . . . . *Trichophyton rubrum*

85a.   Colony cottony, powdery or granular, with pale
        brownish pigment in the reverse on Sabouraud
        and potato glucose agars; club-shaped
        macroconidia sometimes present; urease and *in
        vitro* hair perforation tests positive; alkaline
        reaction on BCP milk solids glucose agar at 7 days
        . . . . *Trichophyton mentagrophytes*

**Non-dematiaceous fungi producing solitary
aleurioconidia and typically isolated from
deep body sites**

86.   (from 66a) Colony resistant to cycloheximide
        (growth on Mycosel agar) 87

86a.   Colony inhibited by cycloheximide, producing terminal aleurioconidia on a conidiophore with tree-like branching; large chlamydospores often formed at 25°C; arthroconidia often present in large quantities . . . . *Sporotrichum pruinosum*

87.   Colony producing one-celled aleurioconidia with smooth walls 88

87a.   Colony producing one-celled aleurioconidia with rough or warty walls 90

88.   Aleurioconidia or arthroconidia rare on Sabouraud glucose agar; fungus dimorphic, converting to a yeast with multipolar, "satellite" budding on brain-heart infusion agar at 37°C
         . . . . *Paracoccidioides brasiliensis*

88a.   Aleurioconidia numerous or moderately numerous on Sabouraud glucose agar, formed on small conidiophores attached to hyphae at right angles 89

89.   Dimorphic fungus converting into large yeasts (8 - 15 m) budding on a broad base on special media at 37°C; exoantigen or probe test positive for *Blastomyces* . . . . *Blastomyces dermatitidis*

89a.   Fungus producing aleurioconidia able to swell and become transformed into thick-walled adiaspores on Sabouraud glucose agar at 37 - 40°C; budding yeasts absent . . . . *Emmonsia parva*

90.   Colony producing unicellular macroconidia, 7 - 15 m, with protuberant, tuberculate warts, as well as microconidia with more or less roughened walls; dimorphic fungus converting to a small budding yeast (2 - 5 m) on appropriate media at 37°C; exoantigen or probe test positive for *Histoplasma* . . . . *Histoplasma capsulatum*

90a. Colony producing large, rough-walled conidia resembling those of *Histoplasma*; microaleurioconidia absent; not converting to a yeast phase at 37°C; exoantigen or probe tests for *Histoplasma* negative
.... *Sepedonium* or *Chrysosporium*

91. (from 65a). Unicellular microconidia accompanied by bi- or multicellular macroconidia; macroconidia slightly or distinctly curved, with a foot cell at the base .... *Fusarium*

91a. Conidia strictly unicellular 92

92. Blastoconidia produced sympodially on short denticles formed at the tip of an erect conidiophore or along the sides of a zigzag conidiophore 93

92a. Phialoconidia produced in sticky masses 95

Non-dematiaceous fungi producing unicellular conidia on short denticles

93. Conidia mainly ovoid, hyaline, formed on denticles grouped into rosettes; brown secondary conidia formed individually along the sides of hyphae in older colonies; a dimorphic fungus converting to a yeast phase on brain-heart infusion agar at 37°C .... *Sporothrix schenckii*

93a. Conidia formed on a conidiogenous cell which is swollen at the base and thinly zigzagging at the tip; yeast phase absent 94

94. Colony white; conidiogenous cells often in compact clusters .... *Beauveria*

94a. Colony yellowish, cinnamon, or purple; conidiogenous cells produced in verticils around the conidiophore................. *Tritirachium*

Non-dematiaceous fungi producing phialoconidia in sticky masses

95. (from 92a). Phialides long and narrow (needle-like) 96

95a. Phialides or adelophialides relatively short 97

96. Phialides solitary; colony glabrous or only slightly downy. . . . . *Acremonium*

96a. Phialides grouped in verticils around the conidiophore; colony downy . . . . *Verticillium*

97. Colony glabrous or nearly so, appearing viscous; pink to salmon in colour, sometimes becoming brown; short adelophialides often emerging from the sides of the hyphae . . . . *Lecythophora*

97a. Colony woolly or strongly tufted; phialides formed at the apex of a branched conidiophore
. . . . 98

98. Phialides grouped in brush-like clusters; large masses of viscous conidia accumulate on the upper surfaces of these clusters . . . . . . *Gliocladium*

98a. Phialides fixed at right angles at or near the tips of a much-branched conidiophore network; this network is roughly pyramidal in overall shape
. . . . *Trichoderma*

99. (from 64a). Arthroconidia present. 100

99a. Arthroconidia absent 107

Non-dematiaceous fungi producing arthroconidia

100. Arthroconidia alternate (disjunctor cells present) 101

100a. Arthroconidia simple (disjunctor cells absent). 103

101. Colony sensitive to cycloheximide (no growth on Mycosel); solitary, terminal aleurioconidia present; large round chlamydospores often present at 25°C .... *Sporotrichum pruinosum*

101a. Colony resistant to cycloheximide; terminal conidia resembling arthroconidia; large chlamydospores absent 102

102. Dimorphic fungus growing in tissue or in special media at 40°C as spherules producing endospores; exoantigen or probe test positive for *Coccidioides* .... *Coccidioides immitis*

102a. Fungus not dimorphic (spherule state absent); exoantigens or probe test negative for *Coccidioides* .... *Malbranchea*

103. Colony yeast-like to lightly powdery, growth slow to moderate; arthroconidia predominantly unicellular; budding cells present or absent ... 104

103a. Colony felt-like to very woolly or cottony; growth very rapid; arthroconidia uni- or bicellular ... 105

104. Colony cream, often with waxy and powdery sectors in concentric rings; budding cells and conidiophores absent .... *Geotrichum*

104a. Initial growth yellowish-white, developing sectors of tan or yellowish hyphae; budding cells present in early growth; arthroconidia developing in hyphal sectors and often produced on conidiophores .... *Arthrographis*

105. Arthroconidia produced within the vegetative hyphae; some bicellular arthroconidia present .... *Scytalidium hyalinum*

105a. Unicellular arthroconidia produced terminally, on a conidiophore 106

106.   Extension of hyphae occurs by a budding process;
         arthroconidia produced in chains with
         ramifications; orange to pinkish aerial mycelium
         tending to accumulate on the underside of the lid
         of the Petri plate .... *Chrysonilia*

106a.   Budding process absent; arthroconidia produced
         in whorls or tufts at the apex of an erect
         conidiophore; colony whitish sometimes
         becoming brownish with age ... *Hormographiella*

107.   (from 99a). Conidia bicellular ...... *Trichothecium*

107a.   Conidia strictly unicellular 108

108.   Annelloconidia pyriform to ovoid, with truncate
         bases 109

108a.   Phialoconidia spherical to ovoid
         (no truncate base) 110

109.   Colony cinnamon, conidiophores frequently
         branched .... *Scopulariopsis brevicaulis*

109a.   Colony grey black, conidiophores primarily
         unbranched .... *Scopulariopsis brumptii*

110.   Conidiophores, branched or unbranched, lacking
         a vesicle (a small vesicle of diameter less than
         twice the diameter of the conidiophore may be
         present), lacking a foot cell, supporting phialides
         grouped in tight, brush-like clusters. 111

110a.   Conidiophores long, unbranched, with an apical
         vesicle bearing phialides, and a base with a foot
         cell intercalated into a substrate hypha. 112

111.   Colony powdery, green, blue, grey brown,
         khaki; tips of the phialides with a short neck
         .... *Penicillium*

111a.   Colony rusty, purple, pink, beige or white but
         never green or blue; tips of phialides with an
         elongated neck. .... *Paecilomyces*

33

Aspergillus species

112.   Colony green or greenish at some stage of growth 113

112a.   Colony a colour other than green or greenish 117

113.   Colony bright yellow green; conidiophores colourless and rough-walled . . . . *A. flavus*

113a.   Colony another tint of green; conidiophore smooth walled 114

114.   (also from 12) Mature colonies with a large number of yellow cleistothecia and of hyphae encrusted with yellow and red material . . . . *A. glaucus* group

114a.   Mature colonies lacking yellow cleistothecia and hyphae encrusted red and yellow; cleistothecia, when present, surrounded with hülle cells 115

115.   Undisturbed conidial heads forming compact columns; phialides uniseriate; colonies blue-green to grey-green; good growth at 48°C . . . . *A. fumigatus*

115a.   Undisturbed conidial heads round or columnar, phialides biseriate, hülle cells sometimes present 116

116.   Undisturbed conidial heads columnar, conidiophores brown and less than 300 μm long; hülle cells typically numerous, red cleistothecia sometimes present . . . . *A. nidulans*

116a.   Undisturbed conidial heads round or in loosely coherent columns, conidiophores usually non-pigmented, over 300 μm long; hülle cells rare or absent . . . . *A. versicolor*

117.   (from 112a) Colony black with undisturbed conidial heads round and with biseriate phialides............................ *A. niger*

117a.   Colony cinnamon brown with undisturbed conidial heads columnar and phialides biseriate .... *A. terreus*

Illustrated key

The organisms included in this key are grouped according to morphologic similarities.

The code appearing as a "superscript" alongside the name of each microorganism, indicates the type or types of conidia produced:

> al = aleurioconidia, an = annelloconidia,
> ar = arthroconidia, bl = blastoconidia,
> ph = phialoconidia, po = poroconidia.

The colored bars give an idea of the colors most often observed on the **surface** of the colonies, *with the exception of the dermatophytes (pp.42-43) where they indicate, instead, the color on the **reverse** of the colonies.*

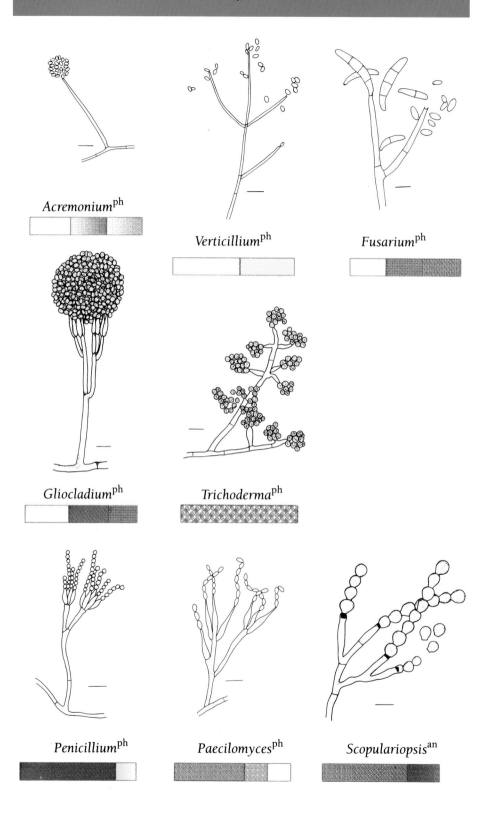

Acremonium[ph]

Verticillium[ph]

Fusarium[ph]

Gliocladium[ph]

Trichoderma[ph]

Penicillium[ph]

Paecilomyces[ph]

Scopulariopsis[an]

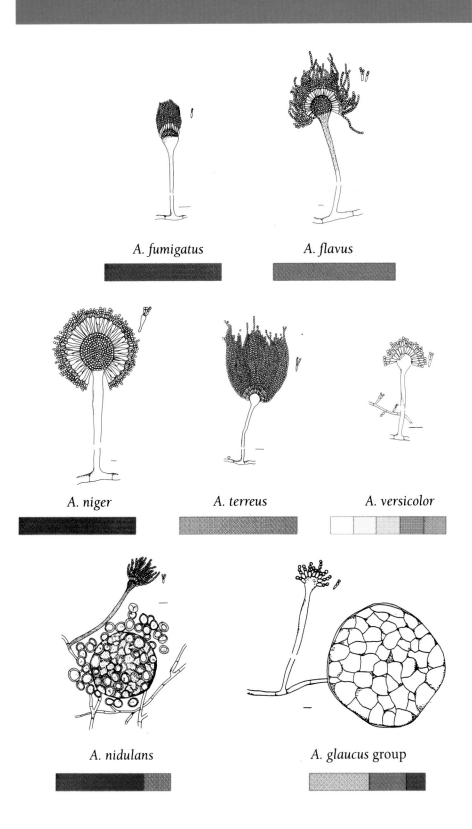

A. fumigatus

A. flavus

A. niger

A. terreus

A. versicolor

A. nidulans

A. glaucus group

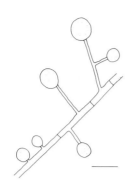

Blastomyces dermatitidis[al]

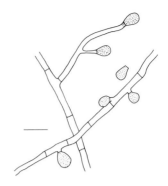

Scedosporium apiospermum[an]

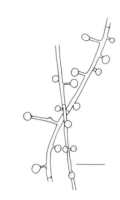

Emmonsia parva[al]

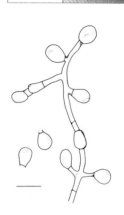

Chrysosporium[al-ar]

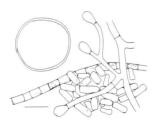

Sporotrichum[al-ar]

40

Plate IV. **Miscellaneous fungi: conidia uni- or bicellular (aleurio[al], blasto[bl], phialo[ph])**

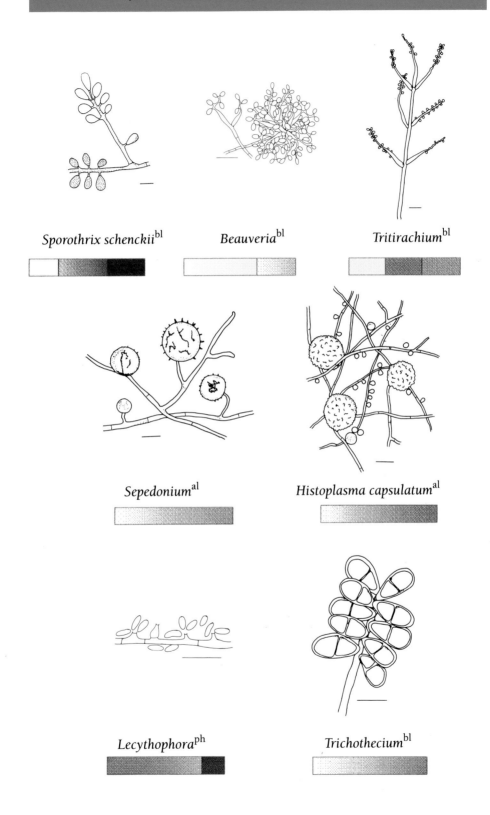

Sporothrix schenckii[bl]

Beauveria[bl]

Tritirachium[bl]

Sepedonium[al]

Histoplasma capsulatum[al]

Lecythophora[ph]

Trichothecium[bl]

41

Plate V. *Epidermophyton* and *Microsporum* species: conidia uni- or multicellular (aleurio)

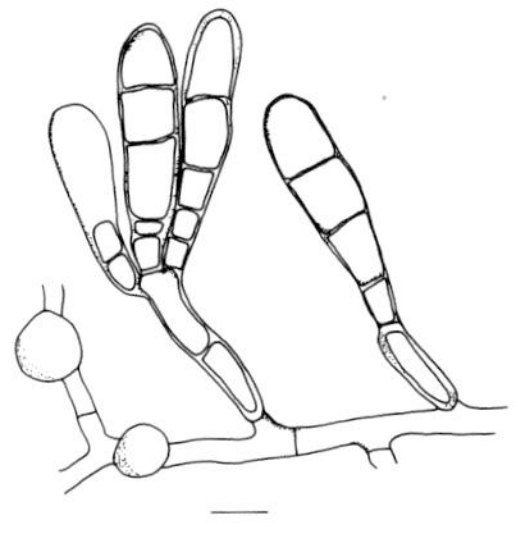

E. floccosum

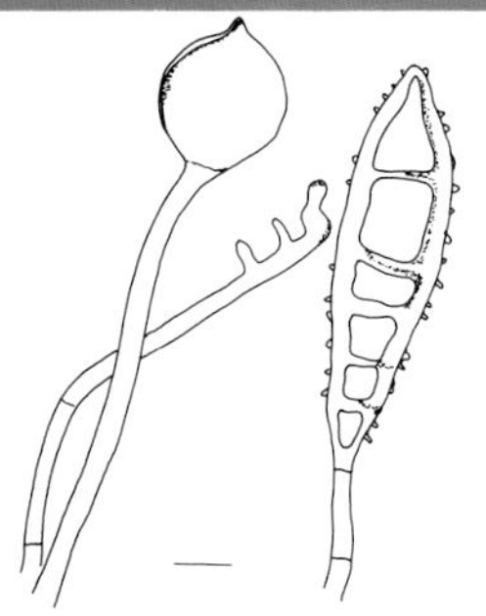

M. audouinii *

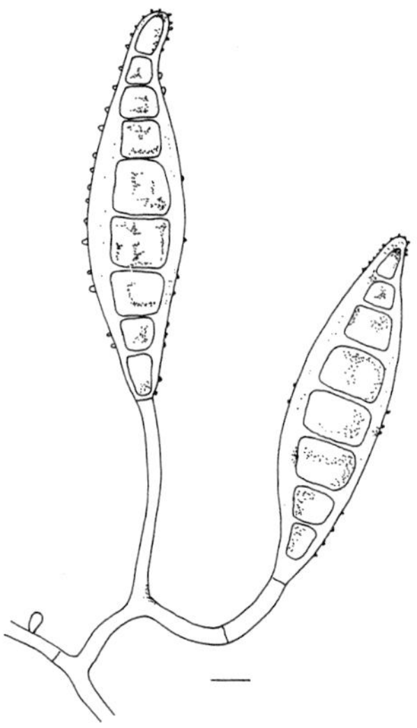

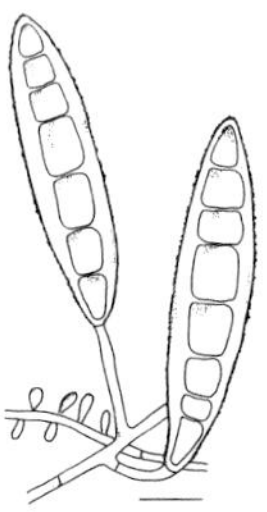

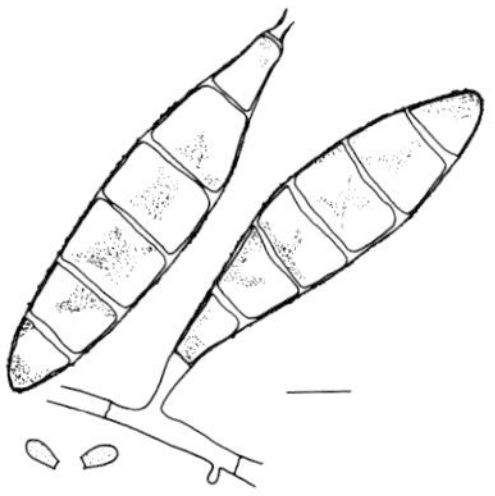

M. gypseum

M. canis

M. cookei

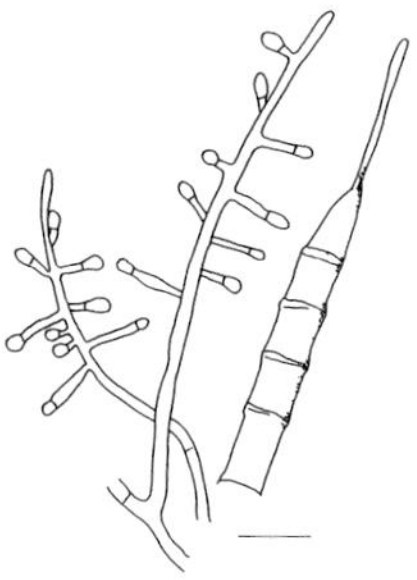

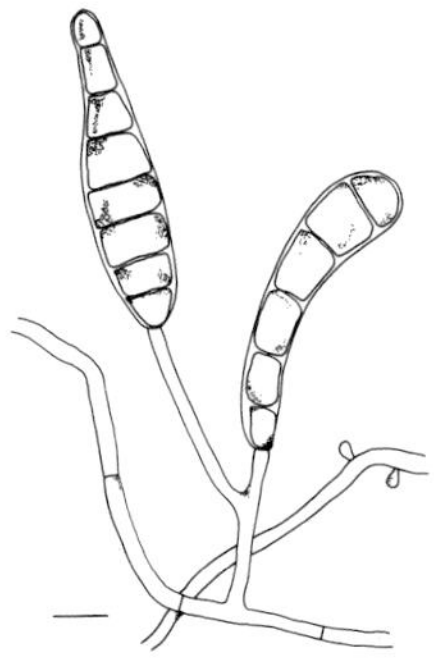

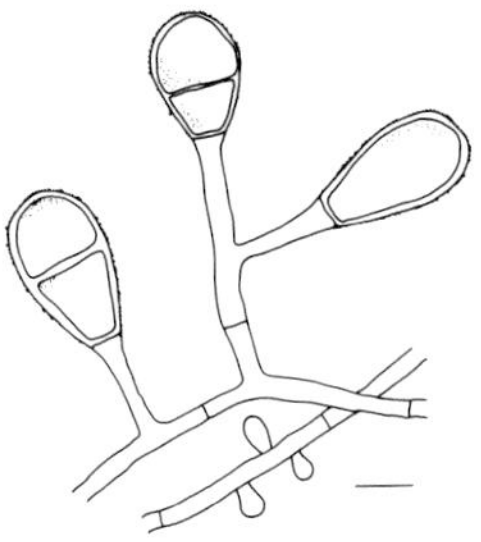

M. persicolor

M. gallinae *

M. nanum

* Macroconidia often absent
Exceptionally, for the dermatophyttes, the colored bars refer to the color on the reverse of the colony.

Plate VI. **_Trichophyton_ species: conidia uni- or multicellular (aleurio)**

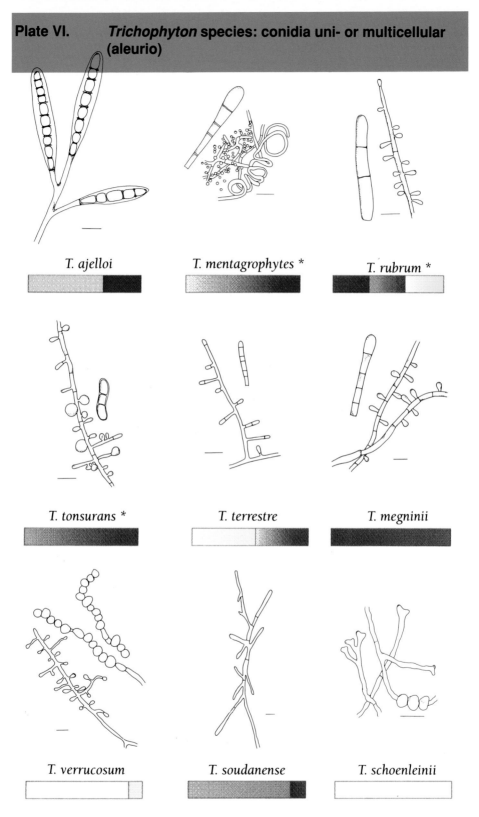

T. ajelloi

T. mentagrophytes *

T. rubrum *

T. tonsurans *

T. terrestre

T. megninii

T. verrucosum

T. soudanense

T. schoenleinii

* Macroconidia often absent

Exceptionally, for the dermatophyttes, the colored bars refer to the color on the reverse of the colony.

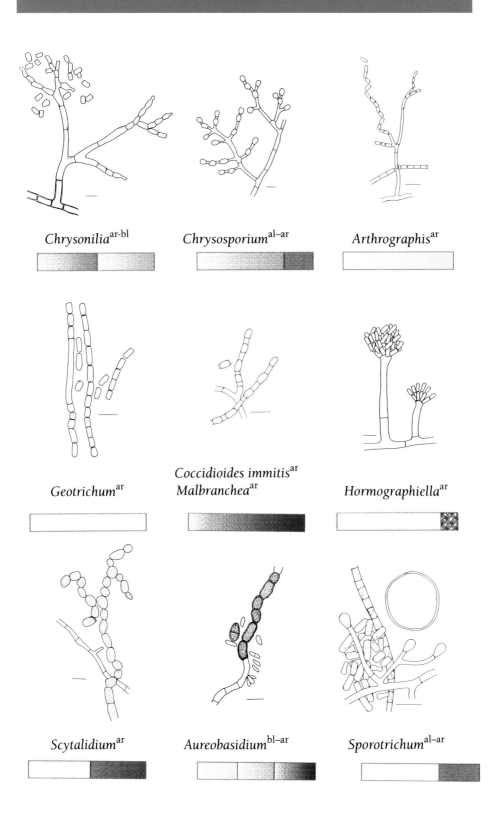

Chrysonilia[ar-bl]

Chrysosporium[al–ar]

Arthrographis[ar]

Geotrichum[ar]

Coccidioides immitis[ar]
Malbranchea[ar]

Hormographiella[ar]

Scytalidium[ar]

Aureobasidium[bl–ar]

Sporotrichum[al–ar]

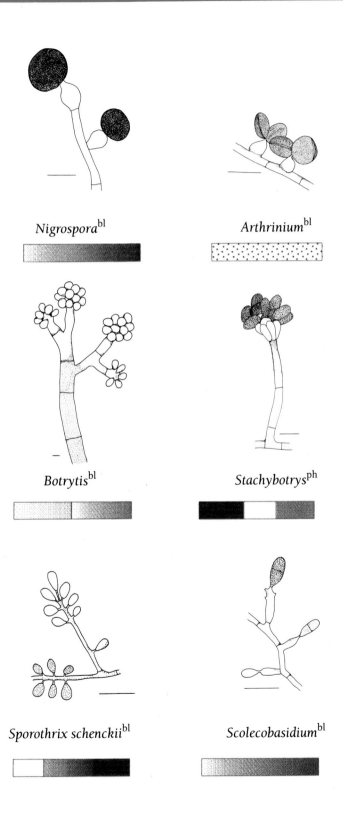

Nigrospora[bl]

Arthrinium[bl]

Botrytis[bl]

Stachybotrys[ph]

Sporothrix schenckii[bl]

Scolecobasidium[bl]

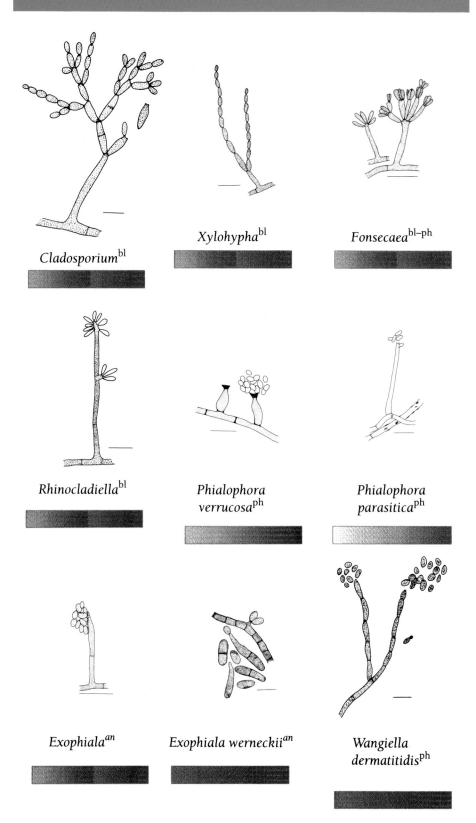

Cladosporium[bl]

Xylohypha[bl]

Fonsecaea[bl-ph]

Rhinocladiella[bl]

Phialophora verrucosa[ph]

Phialophora parasitica[ph]

Exophiala[an]

Exophiala werneckii[an]

Wangiella dermatitidis[ph]

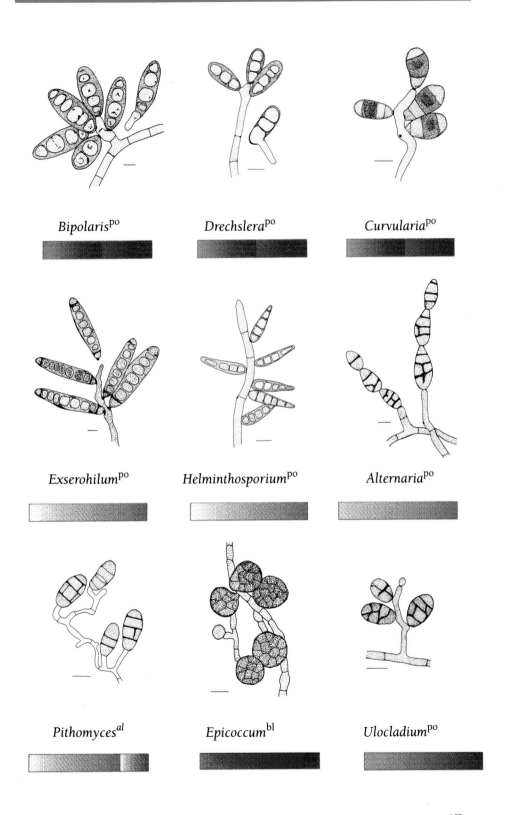

Bipolaris^po^

Drechslera^po^

Curvularia^po^

Exserohilum^po^

Helminthosporium^po^

Alternaria^po^

Pithomyces^al^

Epicoccum^bl^

Ulocladium^po^

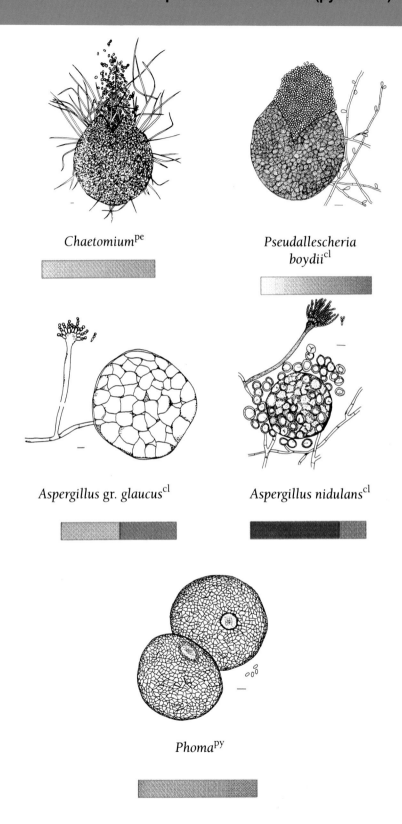

Chaetomium^{pe}

Pseudallescheria boydii^{cl}

Aspergillus gr. glaucus^{cl}

Aspergillus nidulans^{cl}

Phoma^{py}

48

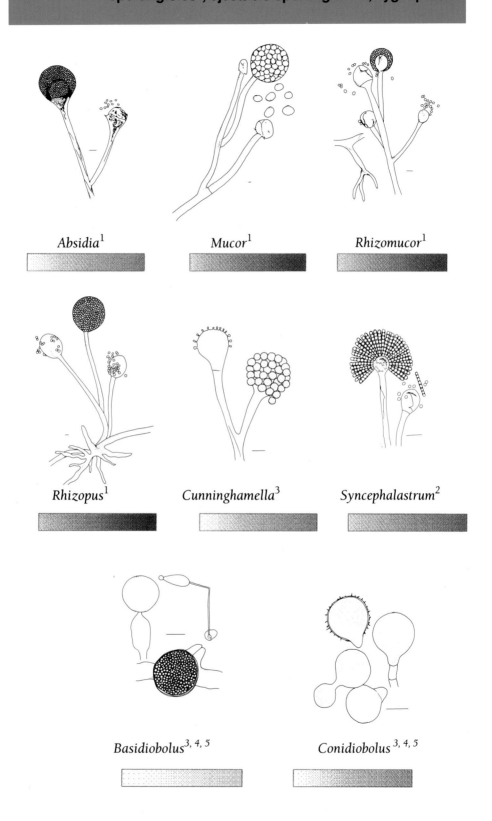

Absidia[1]

Mucor[1]

Rhizomucor[1]

Rhizopus[1]

Cunninghamella[3]

Syncephalastrum[2]

Basidiobolus[3, 4, 5]

Conidiobolus[3, 4, 5]

Descriptions

Growth rate

The growth rate is determined by measuring the diameter of colonies grown at 25°C for 7 days on the media mentioned below, under the heading "Macroscopic and microscopic descriptions":

- very rapid growth: diameter ≥ 9 cm
- rapid growth: diameter between 3 and 9 cm
- moderately rapid: diameter between 1 and 3 cm
- slow growth: diameter between 0,5 and 1 cm
- very slow growth: diameter ≤ 0,5 cm

Macroscopic and microscopic descriptions

The descriptions are based on cultures grown at 25°C on potato glucose agar, with the exception of the dermatophytes and the *Aspergillus* species, cultivated respectively on Sabouraud glucose agar and Czapek-Dox agar.

Remarks

The remarks under each description summarize the principal characteristics of each genus or species described and outline the criteria used for avoiding confusion with similar organisms.

Line drawings

Drawings have been produced at various magnifications, but all are accompanied by a scale bar indicating 10 micrometers. Dense stippling indicates the presence of brown, grey, or black pigment in the cell walls of the dematiaceous fungi.

Photographs

The majority of photographs were taken with a Leitz Ortholux phase contrast microscope equipped with an Orthomat camera attachment. Scale bars represent 10 micrometers or, where specified, 100 micrometers. Colonies were photographed after 7 days of incubation at 25°C on Sabouraud glucose agar or potato glucose agar, according to the fungus grown. The photographs represent not only the color and texture of colonies, but also the growth rate of typical strains.

Absidia van Tieghem, 1876

Pathogenicity: *Absidia corymbifera* is among the recognized agents of zygomycosis. Although this species is most commonly implicated in opportunistic pulmonary invasions, infections of the skin, the meninges, and the kidneys have also been reported, primarily in the immunocompromised patient. *A. corymbifera* occasionally causes mycotic abortion in the cow.

Ecology: most *Absidia* species are cosmopolitan and principally isolated from soil and decaying vegetation.

Colony appearance:
- rapid growth;
- wooly texture;
- color grey on surface, reverse uncolored.

Microscopic features:
- hyphae large, aseptate or with few adventitious septa;
- sporangiophores branched, with a funnel-shaped swelling (apophysis) beneath the sporangium;
- sporangia pyriform;
- rhizoids often few in number, situated on stolons between the sporangiophores.

Remarks: *Absidia* is distinguished from *Mucor*, *Rhizomucor* and *Rhizopus* by its sporangiophores incorporating a well developed apophysis. It produces rhizoids and stolons, but these are often rare or difficult to discern. *Apophysomyces elegans* resembles *A. corymbifera* but has white colonies and does not sporulate on media routinely used in medical mycology. Among the *Absidia* species, *A. corymbifera* is the only recognized pathogen. It is a thermophilic species with a growth rate significantly more rapid at 37°C than at 25°C, and it is able to grow at temperatures up to 48 -52°C. Most other *Absidia* species are unable to grow at 37°C.

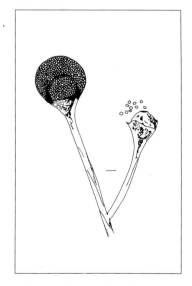

Figure 5.1 *Absidia* sp.

Bibliography:
Domsch, Gams, Anderson, 1980
Kwon-Chung, Bennett, 1992
Scholer, Müller, Schipper, 1983

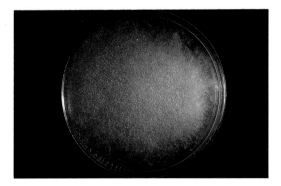

Figure 5.2   *Absidia corymbifera.*
Potato glucose agar,
25°C, 7 days.

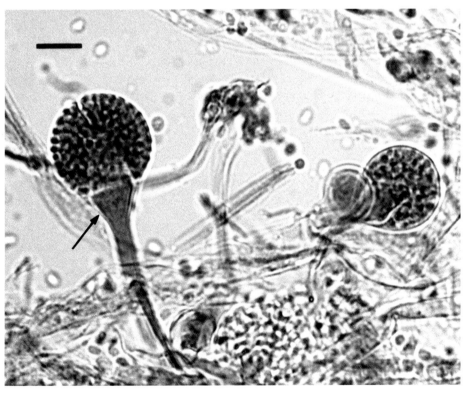

Figure 5.3   *Absidia corymbifera.* Pyriform sporangium with well developed
apophysis↑.

Acremonium Link, 1809

= *Cephalosporium* (Corda, 1839)

Pathogenicity: occasionally a cause of white grain mycetoma. In addition to some cases of onychomycosis, *Acremonium* is also reported from rare cases of keratitis, endophthalmitis, endocarditis, and meningitis, mainly in the immunocompromised patient.

Ecology: cosmopolitan, isolated from soil and plant debris.

Colony appearance:
- moderately rapid growth;
- texture glabrous to lightly downy, sometimes powdery;
- color white, pale grey, or pale pink on the surface; reverse pale.

Microscopic features:
- hyphae septate, hyaline;
- phialides solitary, long and narrow, typically with a septum at the base and a scarcely visible collarette at the apex;
- conidia oblong to ovoid, unicellular (rarely bicellular), often accumulating in heads at the apices of the phialides or occasionally in chains.

Remarks: *Acremonium* produces glabrous to lightly downy colonies with diameters rarely greater than 2 cm at 7 days of incubation. It is important to avoid confusing *Acremonium* with certain isolates of *Fusarium* which do not produce macroconidia, and also with certain *Verticillium* species which produce mostly solitary phialides, with few phialides in verticils. These two groups of isolates normally differ from *Acremonium* either by manifesting faster rates of growth, or by producing deeply wooly colonies. One group of *Acremonium* species, previously referred to as the genus *Gliomastix*, have olive green to greenish black colonies. Unlike *Lecythophora* and *Phialemonium*, *Acremonium* species produce phialides the majority of which are long, narrow, and septate at the base.

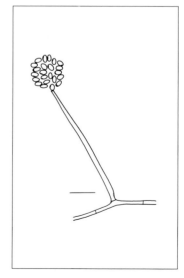

Figure 6.1   *Acremonium sp.*

Bibliography:
Domsch, Gams, Anderson, 1980
Gams, 1971
Gams, McGinnis, 1983
Kwon-Chung, Bennett 1992

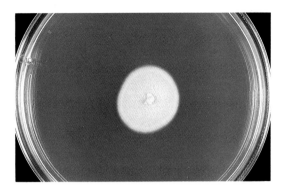

Figure 6.2   *Acremonium kiliense.*
Potato glucose agar,
25°C, 7 days.

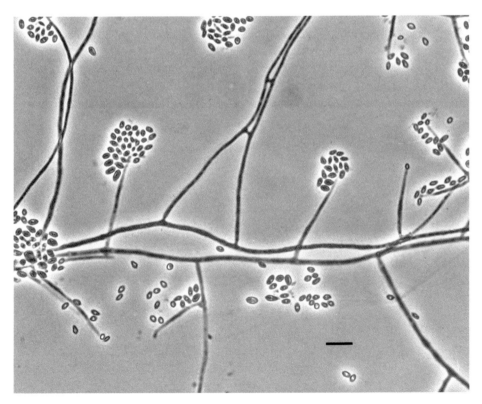

Figure 6.3   *Acremonium kiliense.* Oblong conidia accumulating at the apices
of narrow phialides.

Alternaria Nees, 1816

Pathogenicity: occasional agents of onychomycosis, of ulcerated cutaneous infection, and of chronic sinusitis. Rare cases of deep infection have also been reported in the immunocompromised patient.

Ecology: cosmopolitan, predominantly isolated from plants, either as pathogens or as saprobes, and from soil.

Colony appearance:
- rapid growth;
- texture downy to wooly;
- color pale grey to olive brown on the surface, reverse brown to black.

Microscopic appearance:
- hyphae septate, pigmented brown;
- conidiophores brown, septate, simple or branched, not or scarcely geniculate;
- conidia (poroconidia) brown, muriform, ovoid or obclavate, with an elongated, beak-like apical cell, often in chains, sometimes solitary.

Remarks: *Alternaria* can usually be distinguished from *Ulocladium* by its obclavate conidia with a beak at the apex. Its conidiophores are comparatively less geniculate than those of *Ulocladium*, and its conidia are typically in chains, while those of *Ulocladium* are mostly formed singly or only in very short chains. *Pithomyces*, unlike *Alternaria* does not produce conidia in chains.

Bibliography:
de Bièvre, 1991
de Hoog, 1983
McGinnis, 1980
Domsch, Gams, Anderson, 1980

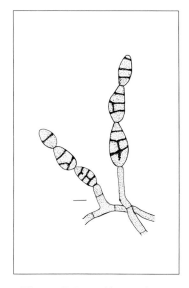

Figure 7.1   *Alternaria* sp.

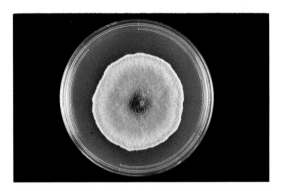

Figure 7.2   Potato glucose agar,
25°C, 7 days.

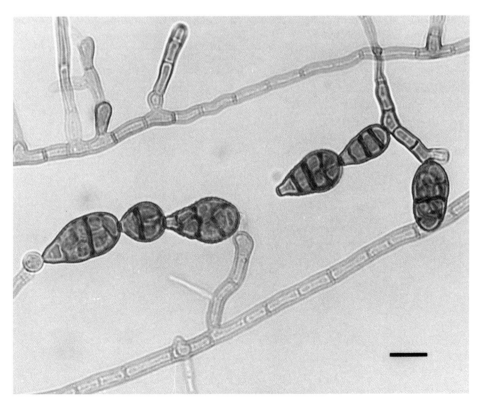

Figure 7.3   *Alternaria* sp. Obclavate, muriform conidia in chains.

Arthrinium Kunze, 1817

Pathogenicity: no cases of infection are reported in humans or animals.

Ecology: cosmopolitan, isolated mainly from decomposing plant material or from soil.

Colony appearance:
- rapid growth;
- texture wooly to cottony;
- color white, spotted with brown on the surface; reverse pale.

Microscopic appearance:
- hyphae septate, hyaline;
- conidiogenous cells pale, short or elongate, more or less inflated at the base;
- conidia brown, lens or lentil shaped, with an equatorial germ slit, formed in dense clusters.

Remarks: *Arthrinium* species are contaminants occasionally encountered in the clinical laboratory. They can be differentiated from *Stephanosporium* by their conidia in clusters rather than in chains. Isolates which are slow to sporulate can be distinguished from dermatophytes and dimorphic pathogens by their sensitivity to cycloheximide.

Bibliography:
Domsch, Gams, Anderson, 1980

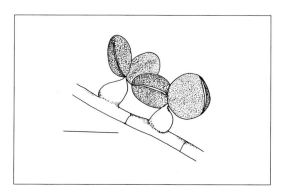

Figure 8.1   *Arthrinium* sp.

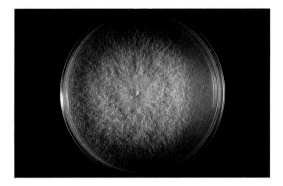

Figure 8.2   Potato glucose agar,
25°C, 7 days.

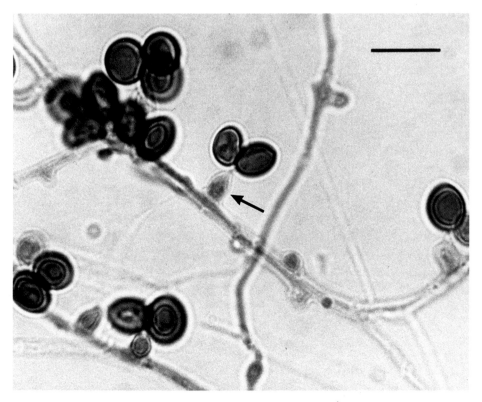

Figure 8.3   *Arthrinium* sp. Inflated conidiogenous cell[↑] and cluster of brown
lentil-shaped conidia.

Arthrographis Cochet ex Sigler and Carmichael, 1976

Pathogenicity: occasionally isolated from respiratory secretions of patients with chronic pulmonary diseases, but no connection with a pathogenic role has yet been elucidated.

Ecology: cosmopolitan, isolated from soil and from compost.

Colony appearance:
- slow to rapid growth;
- texture glabrous becoming velvety;
- color pale yellow on the surface and the reverse.

Microscopic appearance:
- hyphae septate, hyaline;
- conidiophores hyaline, simple or branched;
- arthroconidia formed at the tips of conidiophores or intercalary in the hyphae;
- aleurioconidia sometimes present, mostly on the submerged hyphae;
- yeast cells often present in young colonies, upon primary culture.

Remarks: *Arthrographis* is distinguished from *Geotrichum* and *Scytalidium* by the presence of definite conidiophores. In contrast to *Oidiodendron*, the conidiophores and conidia do not contain grey pigment. Isolates maintained for long periods in the laboratory have a tendency to degenerate; the conidiophores become rare while simple, intercalary arthroconidia become increasingly common. *Arthrographis kalrae* is the species most frequently seen in the clinical laboratory. The presence of yeast cells and growth at 45°C are typical of this species and may aid in its identification.

Bibliography:
McGinnis, 1980
Sigler, 1983

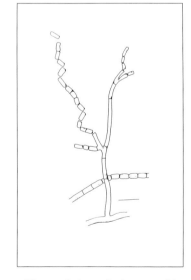

Figure 9.1   *Arthrographis* sp.

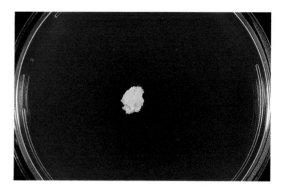

Figure 9.2　*Arthrographis kalrae.*
Potato glucose agar,
25°C, 7 days.

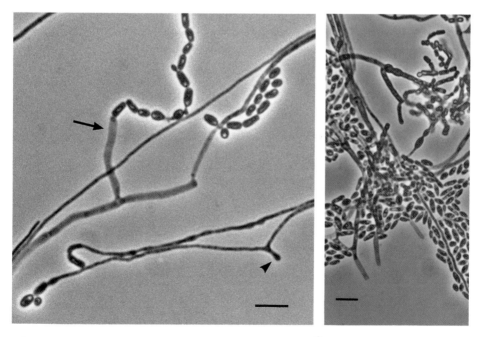

Figure 9.3　*Arthrographis kalrae.* A, Conidiophore[↑] with chains of
arthroconidia; aleurioconidium▲. B, Yeast cells.

61

Aspergillus

Micheli ex Link, 1809

Pathogenicity: at present, some twenty species of *Aspergillus* have been recognized as opportunistic pathogens. Among these, *Aspergillus fumigatus* remains the species most frequently implicated, followed by *Aspergillus flavus* and *Aspergillus niger*. In humans, the most common forms of aspergillosis are pulmonary in nature, although other deep infections are also encountered, particularly in the immunocompromised patient. Numerous outbreaks of disseminated aspergillosis cases have been recorded in neutropenic patients in conjunction with hospital renovation projects. *Aspergillus* species are a frequent cause of respiratory infection in birds; they are also occasionally a cause of mycotic abortion in certain mammals, in particular cattle and sheep.

Ecology: cosmopolitan, saprobic fungi of soils (especially cultivated soils) and decomposing plant material. Airborne contaminants frequently encountered in the clinical mycology laboratory.

Remarks: *Aspergillus* is easily recognized by its conidiophores terminating in an apical vesicle and, at the opposite end, in a basal foot cell inserted into the supporting hyphae. Phialides are attached directly to the vesicle (uniseriate) or on an intervening cell called a metula (biseriate); these structures may cover the entire surface of the vesicle (radiate head) or may be localized primarily on the upper surface (columnar head); conidia are in chains. The identification of species or species groups depends primarily on colony color and the form of conidial heads. The appearance of the species commonly isolated in the clinical laboratory is normally typical on Sabouraud glucose agar or potato glucose agar. Nonetheless, in reference works, descriptions are often of colonies grown on Czapek-Dox agar.

Bibliography:
Domsch, Gams, Anderson, 1980
Kwon-Chung, Bennett, 1992
Raper, Fennell, 1973
Samson, 1979
Samson, Pitt, 1990

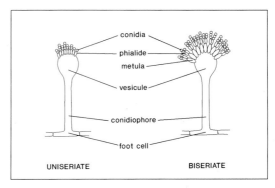

Figure 10.   *Aspergillus* sp. Uniseriate and biseriate aspergillary heads.

Table II. *Aspergillus*: characteristics of species treated.

Species	Colony color surface/reverse	Conidial head	Conidio-phore	Phialides	Other characteristics
A. flavus	yellow green/ yellow, brownish		rough, colorless	uniseriate and biseriate	sclerotia sometimes present
A. fumigatus	grey green, blue green/ yellowish		smooth, colorless or greenish	uniseriate	good growth at 48°C
A. glaucus group	green and yellow/ yellowish, brown		smooth, colorless	uniseriate	yellow to orange cleistothecia present
A. nidulans	green, buff/ purplish red, olive		smooth, brown	biseriate	round hülle cells and red cleistothecia usually present
A. niger	black/ white, yellowish		smooth, colorless or brown	biseriate	
A. terreus	brown cinnamon/ yellowish brown		smooth, colorless	biseriate	round, solitary aleurioconidia, produced directly on hyphae
A. versicolor	white, buff, yellow, pink, pale green/ white, yellow, purplish red		smooth, colorless	biseriate	round hülle cells sometimes present

Aspergillus flavus   Link, 1809

Pathogenicity: an occasional agent of pulmonary or disseminated infection in the immunocompromised patient. Cases of sinusitis and onychomycosis have also been reported. In animals, it may be the agent of respiratory infections of birds.

Ecology: cosmopolitan, isolated mainly from plants and soil. Known especially for its aflatoxins produced in certain foodstuffs such as peanuts.

Colony appearance:
- rapid growth;
- texture downy to powdery;
- color yellow green on the surface; reverse pale or yellowish.

Microscopic appearance:
- conidial heads mostly radiate, with conidial masses splitting into blocky columns at maturity;
- conidiophores with roughened walls, especially near the vesicle;
- phialides uniseriate and biseriate;
- conidia round, rough walled, in chains;
- brown sclerotia produced in some isolates.

Remarks: *A. flavus* is distinguished from other species of *Aspergillus* by its brilliant yellow green colonies and by its typically rough-walled conidiophores.

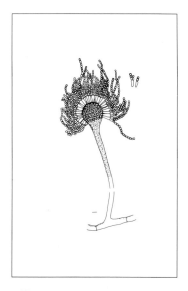

Figure 11.1   *Aspergillus flavus.*

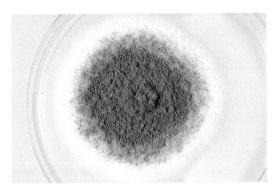

Figure 11.2   Sabouraud glucose agar, 25°C, 7 days.

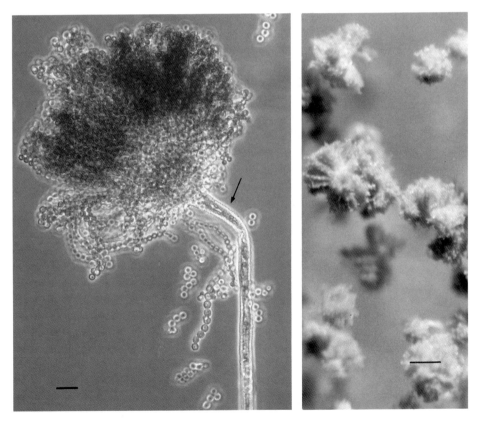

Figure 11.3   *Aspergillus flavus.* A, Conidial head supported by a rough-walled↑ conidiophore. B, Radiate heads with conidial masses splitting into columns at maturity (dissecting microscope, bar = 100 μm).

Aspergillus fumigatus

Fresenius, 1863

Pathogenicity: the most frequently isolated agent of aspergillosis in humans. It may cause pulmonary, nasal, ocular, cerebral, bone, cardiovascular, and organ infections, particularly in the immunocompromised patient. *A. fumigatus* is also a cause of mycotic abortion in the cow and of respiratory infections in fowl.

Ecology: cosmopolitan, thermotolerant, isolated mainly from compost, from soil, and from plant material. One of the most common aspergilli in nature, growing mainly in warm habitats.

Colony appearance:
- rapid growth;
- texture downy to powdery;
- color blue-green to grey green on the surface; reverse pale or yellowish.

Microscopic appearance:
- conidial heads in the form of compact columns;
- conidiophores smooth-walled, often tinted greenish;
- phialides uniseriate, concentrated on the upper surface of the vesicle;
- conidia round, with finely roughened walls, in chains.

Remarks: *A. fumigatus* is distinguished by its blue-green to grey green colonies, its columnar conidial heads, and its uniseriate phialides. Unlike most other medically important species of *Aspergillus*, it develops well at 48°C. An atypical form characterized by downy white colonies lacking any conidial heads is occasionally isolated from cases of aspergilloma or chronic bronchopulmonary colonization. These isolates grow well at 48°C; confirmation of their identity is achieved by stimulating conidial production by culture on potato glucose agar or cornmeal agar at 37°C.

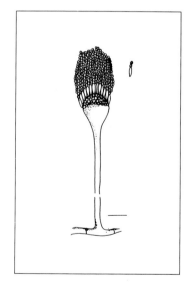

Figure 12.1   *Aspergillus fumigatus.*

66

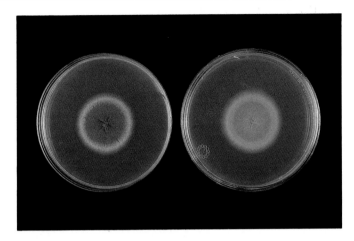

Figure 12.2   Sabouraud glucose agar,
25°C, 7 days.

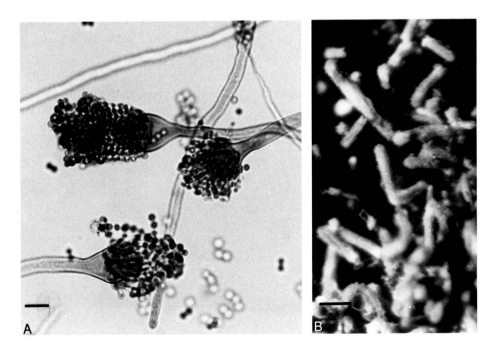

Figure 12.3   *Aspergillus fumigatus.* A, Uniseriate phialides attached to the
upper surface of the vesicle. B, Conidial heads seen as
compact columns (dissecting microscope, bar = 100 µm).

Aspergillus glaucus group

Pathogenicity: only a few cases of pulmonary or disseminated infection have been reported from immunocompromised patients.

Ecology: cosmopolitan, osmophilic, isolated primarily from soil, plants, and house dust.

Colony appearance:
- growth slow to moderately rapid;
- texture downy to powdery;
- color green with yellow sectors on the surface; reverse yellowish to chestnut.

Microscopic appearance:
- conidial heads radiate or loosely columnar;
- conidiophores usually with smooth walls;
- phialides uniseriate;
- conidia ellipsoidal or sometimes round, with wall often roughened, in chains;
- cleistothecia yellow, typically numerous, sometimes more prominent than conidial heads;
- ascospores pale, with or without equatorial crests.

Remarks: the species of *Aspergillus* which belong to the *A. glaucus* group (17 species) are distinguished by the green and yellow coloration of their colonies, with yellow sectors often prominent and corresponding to areas with numerous cleistothecia. Some references discuss these species as members of the genus *Eurotium*, which is the name of the cleistothecial (sexual) state.

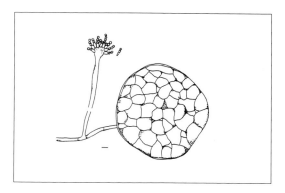

Figure 13.1   *Aspergillus glaucus* group.

Figure 13.2 Sabouraud
glucose agar,
25°C, 7 days.

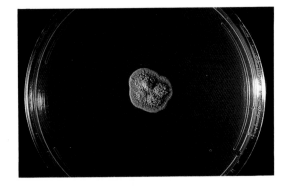

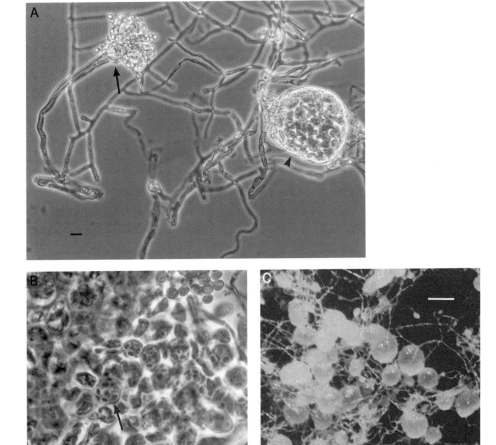

Figure 13.3 *Aspergillus glaucus* group. A, Conidial head[↑] and
cleistothecium▲. B, Ascospores held within an ascus[↑].
C, Cleistothecia (dissecting microscope, bar = 100 μm).

Aspergillus nidulans

(Eidam) Winters, 1884

Pathogenicity: occasionally a cause of pulmonary or disseminated infection in the immunocompromised patient.

Ecology: cosmopolitan, isolated primarily from soil.

Colony appearance:
- growth moderately rapid to rapid;
- texture downy to powdery;
- color dark green or dark olive buff on the surface; reverse purple or olive.

Microscopic appearance:
- conidial heads appearing as short, compact columns;
- conidiophores brown, sinuous, less than 300 μm long;
- phialides biseriate, limited to the upper surface of the vesicle;
- conidia round, with wall more or less roughened, in chains;
- round hülle cells typically present;
- cleistothecia frequently present, reddish in color;
- ascospores red purple, lens shaped, with two equatorial crests.

Remarks: *A. nidulans* is distinguished by its dark green colonies with purple reverse, its brown conidiophores under 300 μm long, its biseriate phialides, and its round hülle cells. Some references list it under the name of the cleistothecial state, *Emericella nidulans*.

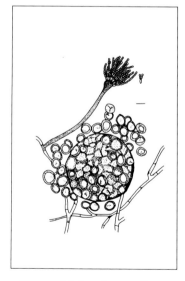

Figure 14.1 *Aspergillus nidulans.*

Figure 14.2 Sabouraud
glucose agar,
25°C, 7 days
(surface/reverse).

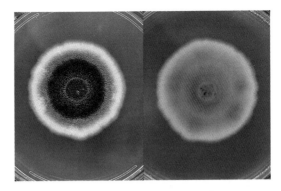

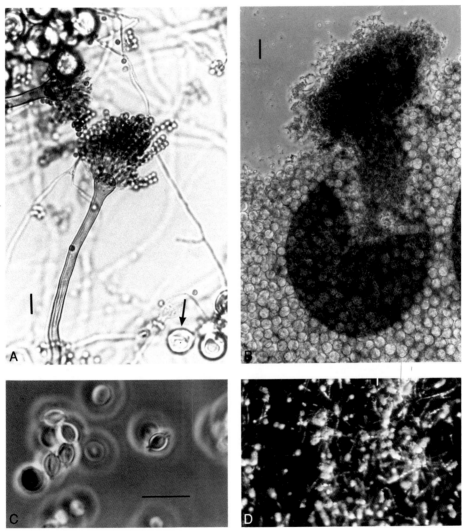

Figure 14.3 *Aspergillus nidulans.* A, Conidial head and round hülle cells ↑.
B, Cleistothecium. C, Ascospores with equatorial crests.
D, Small conidial heads seen as compact columns (dissecting
microscope, bar = 100 μm).

Aspergillus niger

van Tieghem, 1867

Pathogenicity: a frequent agent of aspergilloma. Uncommonly a cause of primary cutaneous, pulmonary, and disseminated infection, particularly in the immunocompromised patient. It is often isolated in cases of chronic otitis where, generally, it colonizes only the outer ear canal without contributing directly to the symptoms.

Ecology: cosmopolitan, isolated mainly from soil and decomposing plant material.

Colony appearance:
- rapid growth;
- texture downy to powdery;
- color white to yellow, becoming black to deep brown on the surface; reverse uncolored or pale yellow.

Microscopic appearance:
- conidial heads radiate, splitting into loosely structured columns in age;
- conidiophores with smooth walls;
- phialides biseriate, covering the entire surface of the vesicle;
- conidia brown, round, rough-walled, in chains.

Remarks: *A. niger* produces a white mycelium which gradually becomes covered with black conidial heads. These heads are radiate and possess biseriate phialides.

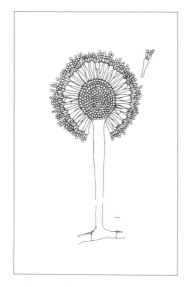

Figure 15.1   *Aspergillus niger.*

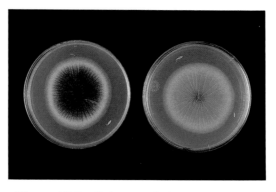

Figure 15.2   Sabouraud glucose agar, 25°C, 7 days.

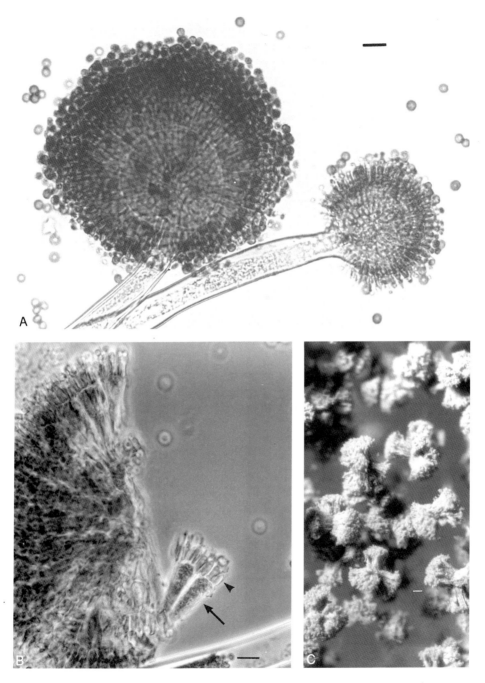

Figure 15.3   *Aspergillus niger*. A, Radiate conidial heads. B, Metulae[↑] and
phialides▲ (conidial head squashed between slide and cover
slip to reveal its biseriate structure). C, Radiate conidial
heads splitting into loose columns (dissecting microscope,
bar = 100 μm).

Aspergillus terreus Thom, 1918

Pathogenicity: occasionally a cause of pulmonary aspergillosis in the immunocompromised host. A few cases of cerebral infection have been reported. Occasionally isolated from outer ear canal colonizations.

Ecology: cosmopolitan, but more common in tropical or subtropical areas. Isolated primarily from soil, compost, and plant material.

Colony appearance:
* rapid growth;
* texture downy to powdery;
* color cinnamon to brown on the surface; reverse pale yellow to brown.

Microscopic appearance:
* conidial heads in the form of compact columns;
* conidiophores hyaline, smooth walled;
* phialides biseriate, limited mainly to the upper part of the vesicle surface;
* conidia in chains, round, smooth walled, brown;
* a second, less conspicuous type of conidia (aleurioconidia) formed singly on the submerged hyphae, round to ovoid, with truncate bases, pale.

Remarks: *A. terreus* is distinguished by its cinnamon to brown colonies, its columnar conidial heads, its biseriate phialides and its solitary aleurioconidia with truncate bases produced directly on the submerged hyphae.

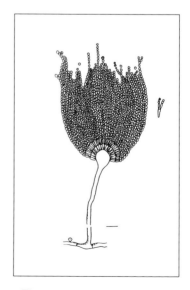

Figure 16.1   *Aspergillus terreus.*

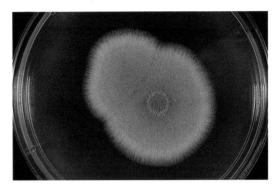

Figure 16.2   Sabouraud glucose agar,
25°C, 7 days.

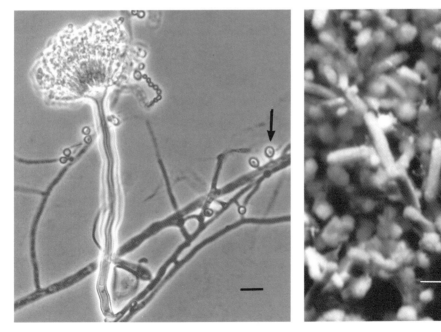

Figure 16.3   *Aspergillus terreus.* A, Conidial head and solitary
aleurioconidia[†] attached directly to a hypha. B, Conidial
heads seen as compact columns (dissecting microscope,
bar = 100 μm).

75

Aspergillus versicolor (Vuillemin) Tiraboschi, 1929

Pathogenicity: rarely a cause of deep infection in humans. Occasionally responsible for cases of onychomycosis.

Ecology: cosmopolitan, commonplace in temperate and colder areas. Isolated primarily from soil and plant materials. Often found in buildings with humidity and ventilation problems.

Colony appearance:
- moderately rapid growth;
- texture downy to powdery;
- color white, yellow, beige, to yellow green or emerald green, sometimes with a clear to wine-red exudate on the surface; reverse pale or yellowish, sometimes orange to purple.

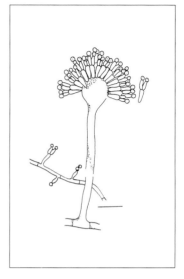

Figure 17.1   *Aspergillus versicolor.*

Microscopic appearance:
- conidial head radiate;

- conidiophores with smooth walls and exceeding 300 μm in length;
- phialides biseriate;
- conidia round, more or less rough-walled, in chains;
- phialides which are solitary or grouped with a few others in a brush-like cluster (reduced conidiogenous structures) are often present;
- hülle cells sometimes present, similar to those of *Aspergillus nidulans*.

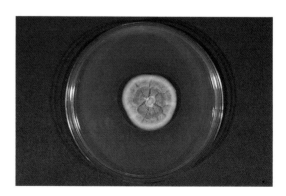

Figure 17.2   *Aspergillus versicolor.* Sabouraud glucose agar, 25°C, 7 days.

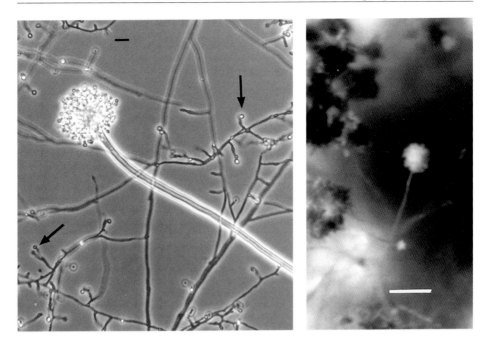

Figure 17.3 *Aspergillus versicolor.* A, Conidial head and reduced conidiogenous structures↑. B, Radiate conidial heads (dissecting microscope, bar = 100 μm).

Remarks: *A. versicolor* is distinguished by its colonies of variable color, usually with a predominantly green tint, its conidiophores measuring over 300 μm and its biseriate phialides. Often, reduced conidiogenous structures are also present. *Aspergillus sydowii*, a species also encountered in the clinical mycology laboratory, is very similar to *A. versicolor* and is distinguished mainly by its deep greenish blue colonies pigmented red brown on the reverse.

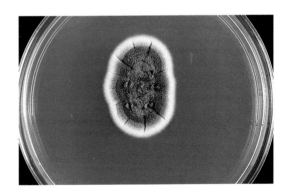

Figure 17.4 *Aspergillus sydowii.* Sabouraud glucose agar, 25°C, 7 days.

Aureobasidium

Viala and Boyer, 1891

Pathogenicity: rarely a cause of keratitis or of cutaneous infection. There have also been a few cases of deep infection in the immunocompromised patient.

Ecology: cosmopolitan, mainly present in temperate zones. The principal habitat is plant leaves, where this fungus is a saprobe and occasionally a phytopathogen. *Aureobasidium pullulans* is frequently isolated as a contaminant of cutaneous surfaces (skin, nails, hair) in humans.

Colony appearance:
- rapid growth;
- mucoid texture;
- color white, pale pink, occasionally pale yellow, becoming brown to black with age; reverse pale.

Microscopic appearance:
- hyphae septate, hyaline, becoming dark brown in age;
- conidiogenous cells little differentiated, intercalary in the hyphae or terminal;
- blastoconidia pale, developing synchronously in tufts;
- chlamydospores or arthroconidia brown, unicellular or bicellular, appearing with age in some isolates.

Remarks: *Aureobasidium* forms mucoid colonies, white or pale pink at first, becoming brown to black with age. It produces hyaline blastoconidia, and brown hyphae which differentiate to form chlamydospores or arthroconidia at maturity. In contrast to *Hormonema*, *Aureobasidium* has blastoconidia appearing synchronously in close tufts, not successively from a single opening.

Bibliography:
Hermanides-Nijhof, 1977
de Hoog, 1983
Kwon-Chung, Bennett, 1992
McGinnis, 1980

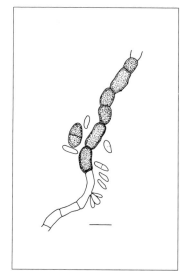

Figure18.1   *Aureo-
basidium
pullulans.*

78

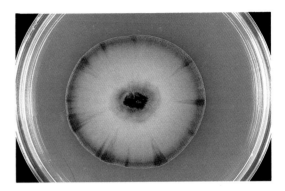

Figure 18.2   *Aureobasidium pullulans.*
Potato glucose agar,
25°C, 7 days.

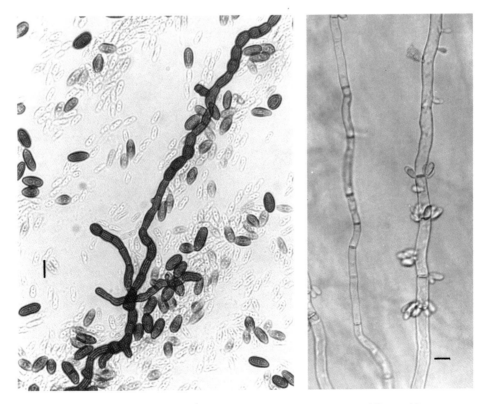

Figure 18.3   *Aureobasidium pullulans.* A, Hyaline blastoconidia and brown
arthroconidia. B, Synchronous blastoconidia (culture by the
Dalmau technique on cornmeal agar).

79

Basidiobolus

Eidam, 1886

Pathogenicity: *Basidiobolus ranarum*, a fungus in the order Entomophthorales, is the etiologic agent of a type of chronic zygomycosis characterized by a thickening of the subcutaneous tissues and adjacent muscles. A few cases of acute zygomycosis similar to cases caused by the Mucorales have also been reported.

Ecology: cosmopolitan, isolated commonly from the dung of amphibians and reptiles and sometimes from plant debris or soil. Despite the broad distribution of the organism, cases of human infection are mostly from Africa, tropical Asia, and south America.

Colony appearance:
- growth moderately rapid (more rapid at 30°C than at 37°C);
- texture waxy; satellite colonies sometimes formed from germination of ejected sporangioles;
- color yellowish to greyish on the surface; reverse pale.

Microscopic appearance:
- hyphae large, 8-20 µm in diameter, more or less septate;
- sporangiophores with inflated apices producing ejectable, unispored sporangioles (ballistospores);
- narrow sporangiophores with adhesive apices producing passively liberated, unispored sporangioles;
- zygospores with conjugation beak.

Remarks: *Basidiobolus* is distinguished from *Conidiobolus* by its zygospores with conjugation beaks. Also, its ejectable sporangioles, once liberated, retain the remnants of the apical portion of the sporangiophore wall at their bases. The sporangiophore, in ejecting the sporangioles, is ruptured by internal turgor pressure leading to a tearing apart of its wall. *Basidiobolus ranarum* (=*Basidiobolus haptosporus*) is the only species recognized as a pathogen.

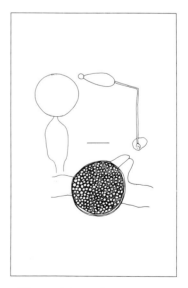

Bibliography:
Kwon-Chung, Bennett, 1992
O'Donnell, 1979

Figure 19.1 *Basidiobolus ranarum.*

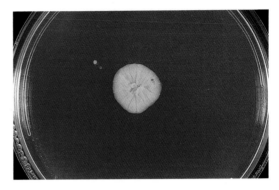

Figure 19.2   *Basidiobolus ranarum.*
Potato glucose agar,
25°C, 7 days.

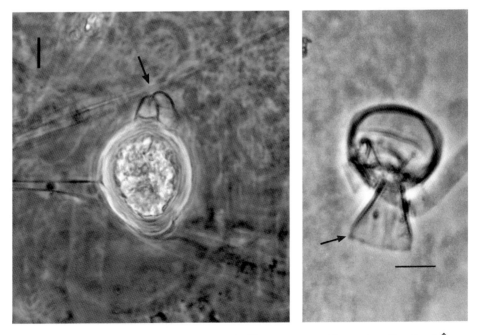

Figure 19.3   *Basidiobolus ranarum.* A, Zygospores with conjugation beak[↑].
B, Ejected sporangioles conserving a fragment of the ruptured
sporangiophore[↑] at its base.

Beauveria Vuillemin, 1912

Pathogenicity: rarely responsible for infection of humans or animals. In addition to some cases of keratitis, a case of pneumonia has also been recorded in an immunocompromised patient. Certain species are important pathogens of insects.

Ecology: cosmopolitan, isolated from soil and from parasitised insects. *Beauveria bassiana* is well known as an agent of muscardine disease of the silkworm.

Colony appearance:
- moderately rapid growth;
- texture cottony to powdery;
- color white becoming pale yellow or pale pink on the surface; reverse pale.

Microscopic appearance:
- hyphae septate, hyaline;
- conidiogenous cells inflated at the base, terminating in a thin, zigzagging filament; these cells often grouped in dense masses;
- conidia hyaline, unicellular, round or oval.

Remarks: *Beauveria* is distinguished by its conidiogenous cells with somewhat inflated bases and zigzagging apices, producing conidia in a sympodial fashion. These cells are minuscule and are often grouped in dense clusters, rendering examination difficult.

Bibliography:
Domsch, Gams, Anderson, 1980
McGinnis, 1980
Rippon, 1988

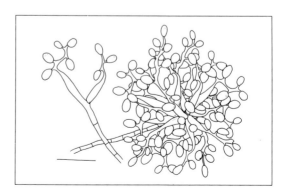

Figure 20.1 *Beauveria bassiana.*

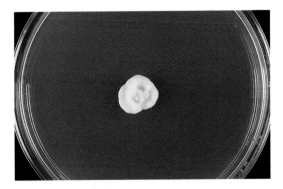

Figure 20.2 *Beauveria bassiana.*
Potato glucose agar,
25°C, 7 days.

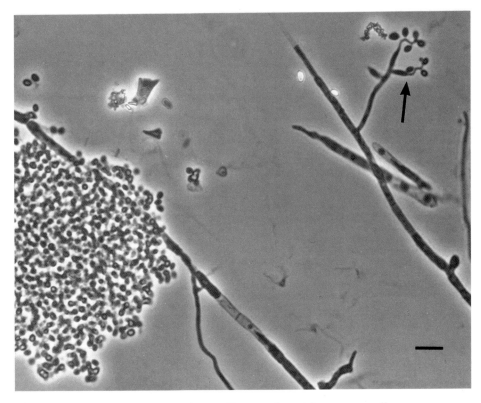

Figure 20.3 *Beauveria bassiana.* Cluster of conidiogenous cells;
conidiogenous cell with inflated base and zigzag apex↑.

Bipolaris

Shoemaker, 1959

Pathogenicity: occasionally the cause of diverse types of phaeohyphomy-cosis, including sinusitis, keratitis, peritonitis, endocarditis, osteomyelitis, meningo-encephalitis, and cutaneous infection; these infections have been rec-ognized in the immunocompromised patient as well as in the normal host.

Ecology: cosmopolitan, although some species are mainly found in tropical or subtropical areas. Saprobes or pathogens of numerous species of plants, par-ticularly Graminae.

Colony appearance:
- rapid growth;
- downy texture;
- color whitish becoming dark olive to black on the surface and reverse.

Microscopic appearance:
- hyphae septate, brown;
- conidiophores brown, geniculate;
- poroconidia brown, fusoid, distoseptate, typically containing 3 to 6 cells; base with a scarcely protuberant hilum;
- germ tubes developing from the terminal cells of the conidium, and growing in the direction of its longitudinal axis.

Remarks: *Bipolaris* is distinguished from *Exserohilum* by its conidia with a scarcely protuberant hilum. The germ tubes of *Bipolaris* are polar and develop in the direction of the long axis of the conidium whereas those of *Drechslera* emerge from any cell of the conidium, perpendicular to the long axis. Unlike the conidia of *Curvularia*, those of *Bipolaris* are distoseptate, that is to say, they are not partitioned from side to side by septa, but instead, their cells are con-tained in sacs which have a wall distinct from the outer wall of the conidium.

Bibliography:
Ellis, 1971
Ellis, 1976
de Hoog, 1983
Kwon-Chung, Bennett, 1992
McGinnis, Rinaldi, Winn, 1986

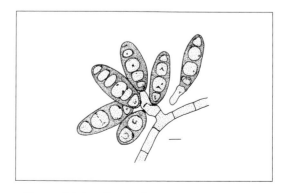

Figure 21.1   *Bipolaris* sp.

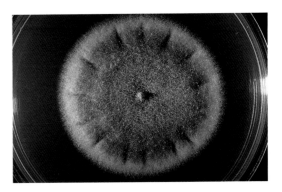

Figure 21.2   *Bipolaris hawaiiensis.*
Potato glucose agar,
25°C, 7 days.

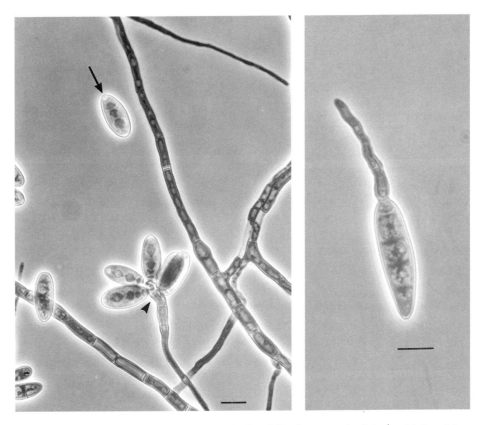

Figure 21.3   *Bipolaris hawaiiensis.* A, Conidiophore geniculate▲ with fusoid,
multiseptate conidia; scarcely protuberant hilum↑. B, Germ
tube developing in the direction of the long axis of the
conidium.

85

Blastomyces dermatitidis   Gilchrist and Stokes, 1898

Pathogenicity: *Blastomyces dermatitidis* is the etiologic agent of blastomycosis, primarily a pulmonary infection which may disseminate to other areas of the body, especially the skin and the bones.

Ecology: rarely isolated from the environment, probably a saprobe of the soil. Endemic zones are mainly found in North America and extend from east central Canada to central America. In the United States, the greatest number of cases are reported from the Mississippi, Ohio and Missouri valleys. A number of cases are also reported from Africa and the Middle East.

DIMORPHIC FUNGUS

Colony appearance:

at 25°C:

- slow to moderately rapid growth;
- texture downy;
- color white to beige on the surface; reverse pale to brownish

at 37°C, on rich medium

- growth slow to moderately rapid;
- texture creamy, granular to verrucose;
- color white to beige.

Microscopic appearance:

at 25°C:

- hyphae septate, hyaline;
- conidiophores short, unbranched;
- conidia hyaline, pyriform, unicellular, terminal, solitary.

at 37°C, on rich medium or in infected tissues:

- yeasts with refractile walls, budding on a broad base.

Remarks: *B. dermatitidis* is a pathogenic fungus which should only be manipulated in culture in a biological safety cabinet in a containment laboratory. It is distinguished from *Chrysosporium* and from *Scedosporium* by its thermal dimorphism characterized by the formation of large yeast cells budding on a broad base when incubated at 37°C on specialised medium. It can also be identified by means of commercial kits, specifically by immunodiffusion (exoantigen) or by hybridization.

Bibliography:
Kwon-Chung, Bennett, 1992
McGinnis, 1980
Rippon, 1988

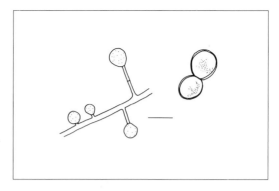

Figure 22.1   *Blastomyces dermatitidis.*

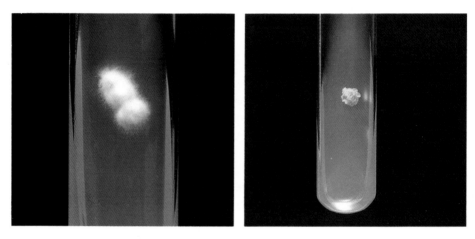

Figure 22.2   A, Mycelial form on Sabouraud glucose agar, 25°C, 7 days.
B, Yeast form on brain heart infusion agar, 37°C, 7 days.

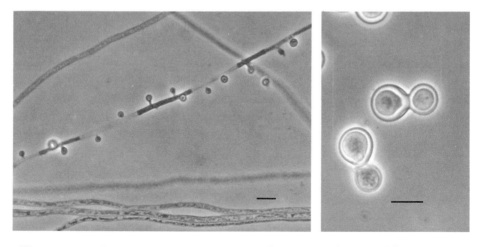

Figure 22.3   *Blastomyces dermatitidis.* A, Solitary, pyriform conidia.
B, Yeasts with refractile wall and broadly based budding.

Botrytis

Micheli ex Persoon, 1801

Pathogenicity: no cases of infection have been recorded in humans or animals.

Ecology: cosmopolitan, but often recorded from regions of humid climate, both temperate and tropical. Saprobes frequently isolated from decaying vegetal matter and facultative pathogens of numerous plants.

Colony appearance:
- growth rapid;
- texture wooly;
- color white becoming grey to brown on the surface; reverse dark.

Microscopic appearance:
- hyphae septate, hyaline to brown;
- conidiophores large, septate, brown, with apical branches terminating in vesicles;
- conidia (blastoconidia) hyaline or pale brown, unicellular, round to oval, formed on denticles on the surface of the vesicles;
- sclerotia or dense pseudoparenchymatous tissue often present.

Remarks: *Botrytis* is distinguished by the production of blastoconidia on the surfaces of vesicles formed at the apices of long, robust brown conidiophores. Also frequently formed are sclerotia or areas of dense pseudoparenchymatous tissue, visible to the naked eye as dark spots on the *surface of the colonies. For optimal sporulation, it is sometimes necessary to incubate the cultures intermittently under an ultraviolet lamp.*

Bibliography:
Domsch, Gams, Anderson, 1980
Hennebert, 1973

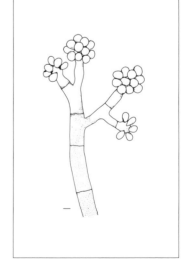

Figure 23.1   *Botrytis* sp.

Figure 23.2   Potato glucose
              agar, 25°C,
              7 days.

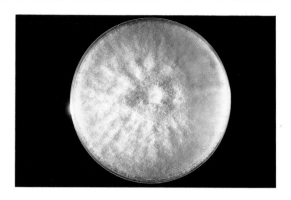

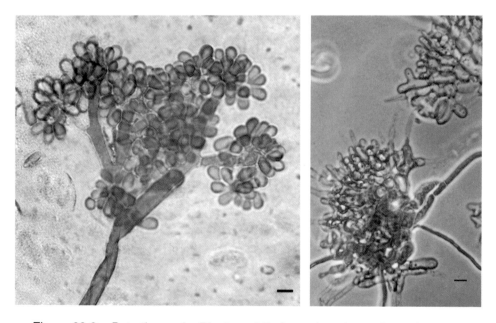

Figure 23.3   *Botrytis* sp. A, Blastoconidia formed on the surface of vesicles
              situated at the apices of long, stout, brown conidiophores.
              B, Pseudoparenchymatous tissue.

Chaetomium Kunze: Fries 1817

Pathogenicity: very uncommonly an agent of onychomycosis or of subcutaneous or deep infection in humans. No cases reported in animals.

Ecology: cosmopolitan, commonly isolated from soil, from decomposing plant materials, especially woody or straw-like materials, as well as from herbivore dung.

Colony appearance:
* rapid growth;
* texture wooly;
* color white becoming grey to olivaceous on the surface; reverse pale yellow to olive brown.

Microscopic appearance:
* hyphae septate, hyaline to pale brown;
* perithecia brown to black, round to ovoid, surrounded by long, undulant, helical or erect, spine-like setae;
* asci evanescent, that is, remaining intact only for a short period after their formation;
* ascospores brown, unicellular, most commonly lemon-shaped.

Remarks: *Chaetomium* is readily recognized by its perithecia enveloped by long brown setae and its brown, lemon-shaped ascospores. The ostiole, or perithecial opening, is often concealed by the density of setae.

Bibliography:
Domsch, Gams, Anderson, 1980
Kwon-Chung, Bennett, 1992

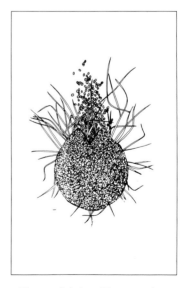

Figure 24.1 *Chaetomium* sp.

90

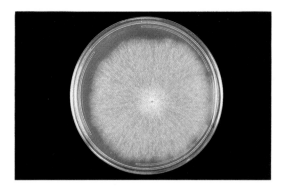

Figure 24.2   Potato glucose agar,
25°C, 7 days.

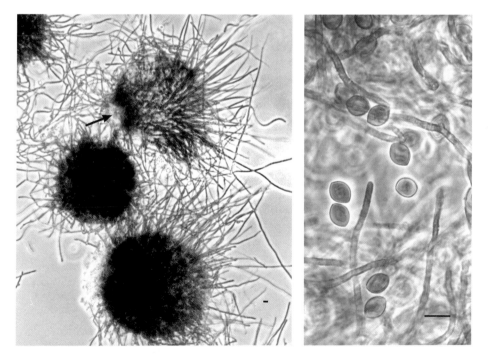

Figure 24.3   *Chaetomium* sp. *Chaetomium* sp. A, Perithecia with long brown
setae; ostiole↑. B, Lemon-shaped ascospores.

91

Chrysonilia von Arx, 1981

= *Monilia* Bonorden, 1851 auct., pro parte (i.e., partially corresponds to the genus *Monilia*, as once defined by some authors). The once broad genus *Monilia*, which long included the species described below, is now restricted to certain plant pathogens seldom seen in the clinical laboratory.
= asexual states of the genus *Neurospora*.

Pathogenicity: no cases of infection have been recorded in humans or animals.

Ecology: cosmopolitan, saprobes of soil.

Colony appearance:
- very rapid growth;
- texture deeply cottony;
- color white, pale pink or pale orange on the surface; reverse pale to orange.

Microscopic appearance:
- hyphae septate, hyaline;
- conidiophores simple or branched;
- arthroconidia hyaline, unicellular, in branching chains which disarticulate easily at maturity;
- blastoconidia produced in chains as part of the process of hyphal extension.

Remarks: *Chrysonilia sitophila* (= *Monilia sitophila*) is a nonpathogenic fungus occasionally isolated in the clinical laboratory. Its white to orange colonies grow aggressively and sporulate abundantly. It is wise to avoid unnecessary manipulation of these colonies as they may cause formidable cross-contamination problems within the laboratory.

Bibliography:
von Arx, 1981
McGinnis, 1980

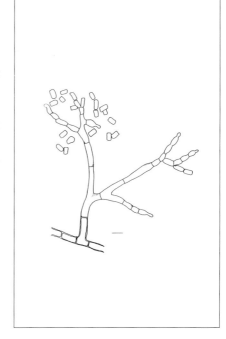

Figure 25.1 *Chrysonilia* sp.

Figure 25.2 *Chrysonilia sitophila.* Potato glucose agar, 25°C, 7 days.

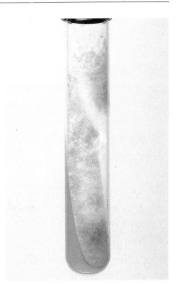

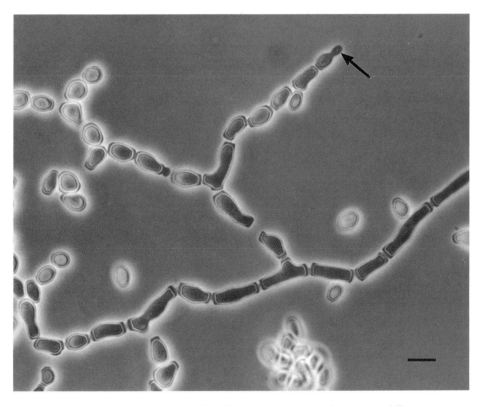

Figure 25.3 *Chrysonilia sitophila.* Branched chains of arthroconidia; blastoconidium↑.

Chrysosporium Corda, 1833

Pathogenicity: although occasional reports of skin and nail infection have been published, the reliability of most of these reports is questionable. One species has been substantiated on rare occasions as an agent of onychomycosis.

Ecology: cosmopolitan, very common saprobes. Many species are keratinophiles.

Colony appearance:
- growth slow to moderately rapid;
- texture powdery to wooly;
- color white, pale yellow or pale brown on the surface; reverse pale to brown.

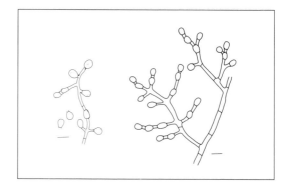

Microscopic appearance:
- hyphae septate, hyaline;
- conidiophores sometimes minimally differentiated from hyphae, sometimes ramified to form tree-like structures;

Figure 26.1 *Chrysosporium* sp.

- conidia (aleurioconidia) hyaline, unicellular, commonly pyriform or club-shaped, solitary or in short chains, formed at the ends of short pedicels or directly on the supporting hyphae;
- arthroconidia most often broader in diameter than the supporting hyphae, intercalated more or less randomly within the conidiogenous hyphae or in short terminal chains of 2 to 3 cells.

Remarks: *Chrysosporium* species are resistant to cycloheximide and may therefore develop on the selective media used for the isolation of dermatophytes. In contrast to the dermatophytes, they often develop conidiophores with branches diverging at 45° angles, unlike the 90°angle at which most dermatophyte microconidia are borne. Many *Chrysosporium* species may produce conidia in short terminal chains, a feature not found in dermatophytes. Species with short terminal chains of conidia grouped in small, tree-like clusters are now often placed in the genus *Geomyces* rather than *Chrysosporium*; these species have been retained in their traditional grouping with *Chrysosporium* here simply because the distinction of the two genera is relatively technical and is best performed by a mycologist. The mold phase of *Blastomyces dermatitidis* is *Chrysosporium*-like, but many *Chrysosporium* species differ by producing arthroconidia, and none transforms into a yeast phase at 37°C. Finally, they differ from *Emmonsia parva* (=*Chrysosporium parvum*) and from *Sporotrichum* by not producing adiaspores at 37-40°C or large chlamydospores at 25°C.

Figure 26.2   Potato glucose
agar, 25°C,
7 days.

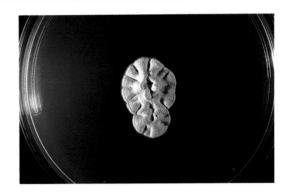

Bibliography:
Domsch, Gams, Anderson, 1980
Kwon-Chung, Bennett, 1992
van Oorschot, 1980

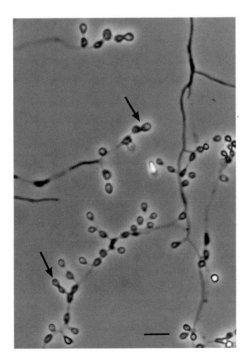 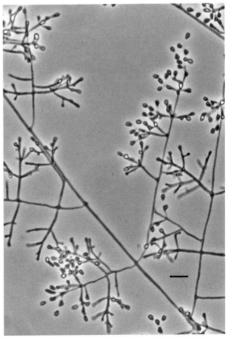

Figure 26.3   *Chrysosporium* sp. A, Terminal conidia in short chain[↑].
B, Branches set at 45° to the main branch.

Cladosporium Link, 1815

Pathogenicity: generally nonpathogenic, with the exception of *Cladosporium carrionii*, an agent of chromoblastomycosis. This is a chronic subcutaneous infection characterized by verrucous lesions and the formation of brown, sclerotic fission cells ("copper pennies") in tissue. It is often confined to a single limb.

Ecology: many species are cosmopolitan fungi of soil, plant debris, and leaf surfaces. *Cladosporium* is very frequently isolated from air, especially during seasons in which humidity is elevated. Infections due to *C. carrionii* are limited to tropical and subtropical regions.

Colony appearance:
- growth slow to rapid;
- texture velvety;
- color olive brown to brownish-black, on the colony surface and on the reverse.

Microscopic appearance:
- hyphae septate, brown;
- conidiophores brown, often septate;
- blastoconidia brown, in very fragile branching chains, bicellular and shield shaped at the base of the chains, unicellular and ellipsoidal to round at the tip; prominent black scars are visible at the points of attachment.

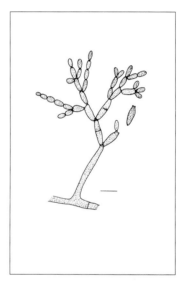

Figure 27.1   *Cladosporium* sp.

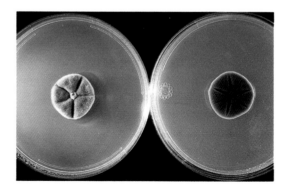

Figure 27.2   *Cladosporium* sp. Potato glucose agar, 25°C, 7 days (surface/reverse).

96

Remarks: the great majority of *Cladosporium* isolates obtained in the clinical laboratory belong to nonpathogenic species incapable of growing at 35-36°C. The presence of conidia in fragile branching chains, with prominent scars at the points of attachment, is characteristic of these species. *C. carrionii* is distinguished by its slow growth, its ability to grow at 35-36°C and sometimes even at 37°C, and its moderately ramified chains of oval, unicellular conidia, more resistant to disarticulation than those of the nonpathogenic species. *Xylohypha bantiana* (*Cladosporium bantianum*) produces long, scarcely branching chains of unicellular conidia and grows at 42-43°C.

Bibliography:
de Hoog, 1983
Domsch, Gams,
  Anderson, 1980
McGinnis, 1980

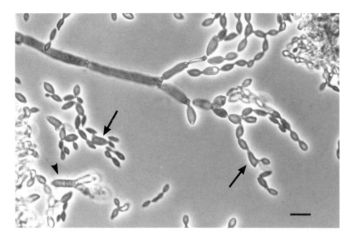

Figure 27.3   *Cladosporium* sp. Shield-shaped conidia↑ with scars at points of attachment; bicellular conidium▲.

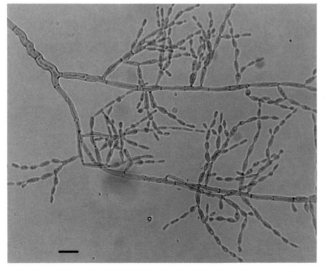
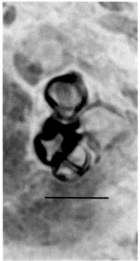

Figure 27.4   *Cladosporium carrionii.* A, Unicellular conidia in strongly ramified chains. B, Sclerotic fission cells in subcutaneous tissues.

Coccidioides immitis Rixford et Gilchrist, 1896

Pathogenicity: *Coccidioides immitis* is the etiologic agent of coccidioi-domycosis, an often benign and transient infection of the respiratory system which in some cases assumes an acute form and may disseminate to infect the skin, the bones, the joints, the liver, and the urogenital and central nervous systems. It is without doubt the most virulent of the pathogenic fungi. Coccidioidomycosis affects both humans and animals.

Ecology: a soil saprobe found principally in certain parts of the southwestern United States and northern Mexico. Some endemic regions are also found in South America. It can be isolated from the microbially depauperate soils of hot, semiarid regions, where its growth is favoured by the low degree of competition from other soil microorganisms.

DIMORPHIC FUNGUS

Colony appearance:

at 25°C and 37°C:
- growth moderately rapid to rapid;
- texture wooly to glabrous;
- color white, sometimes beige, pink, cinnamon, yellow or brown on the surface; reverse pale, sometimes orange, or pale to dark brown.

Microscopic appearance:

at 25°C and 37°C:
- hyphae septate, hyaline;
- conidiophores absent;
- arthroconidia unicellular, rectangular to barrel shaped, often somewhat wider in diameter than the hyphae, alternating with empty cells (disjunctors); freed arthroconidia possess annular frills which are persistent remnants of the wall of the broken disjunctor.

at 42°C on special media or at 37°C in infected tissue:
- spherules (10-80 μm) containing endospores.

Remarks: *Coccidioides immitis* is a dangerous fungus which should only be manipulated in culture in a biological safety cabinet in a containment laboratory. Its alternate arthroconidia with diameter slightly greater than the diameter of the hyphae are liberated by the lysis of the disjunctors and retain an annular frill at the ends. *C. immitis* is distinguished from *Malbranchea* by its capacity to produce spherules in special media at 42°C or in the tissues of animals infected experimentally. Currently, these techniques are little used in the clinical laboratory; they have been replaced by immunodiffusion tests (exoantigen) or by nucleic acid hybridization studies which are both safer and more rapid.

Bibliography:
Huppert, Sun, Rice, 1978
Kwon-Chung, Bennett, 1992
Sigler, Carmichael, 1976
Rippon, 1988

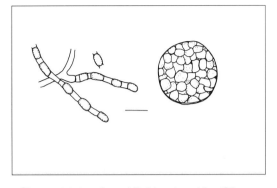

Figure 28.1 *Coccidioides immitis*. Filamentous form and spherule.

Figure 28.2 Sabouraud glucose agar, 25°C, 28 days.

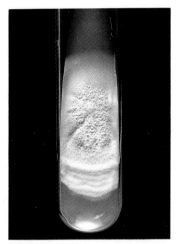

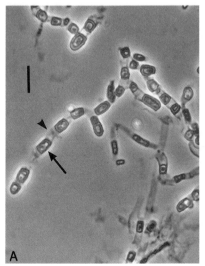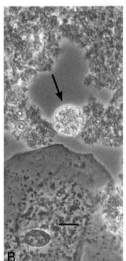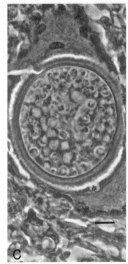

Figure 28.3 *Coccidioides immitis*. A, Alternate arthroconidia[↑] with disjunctors[▲]. B, Spherule[↑] in a sputum specimen. C, Spherule in a tissue section stained with hematoxylin-eosin.

Conidiobolus   Brefeld, 1884

Pathogenicity: fungi of the order Entomophthorales which can cause a type of chronic zygomycosis presenting initially as an infection of the nasal mucous membranes. Recently, some cases of disseminated infection in the immunocompromised host have been reported.

Ecology: cosmopolitan, commonly isolated from humid soils, from decaying plant material or from parasitized insects. The majority of human cases come from tropical and subtropical regions.

Colony appearance:
- very rapid growth;
- satellite colonies formed from ejected sporangioles;
- texture waxy to powdery;
- color white becoming beige to brown on the surface; reverse pale.

Microscopic appearance:
- hyphae broad, more or less septate;
- sporangiophores scarcely differentiated from vegetative hyphae;
- one-spored sporangioles, ejectable (ballistospores), round to pyriform but with a prominent papilla; sporangiole surface smooth or villose, that is, covered with small protuberances. Some sporangioles germinate and produce numerous secondary sporangioles, sometimes forming a crown of sporangioles around themselves.

Remarks: *Conidiobolus*, unlike *Basidiobolus*, possesses sporangiophores with unswollen apices and sporangioles which, once ejected, possess a papilla. *Conidiobolus coronatus* and *C. incongruus* are the two recognized pathogenic species. *C. coronatus* produces villose sporangioles but does not produce zygospores. *C. incongruus*, a homothallic species, produces zygospores without conjugation beaks but does not produce villose sporangioles.

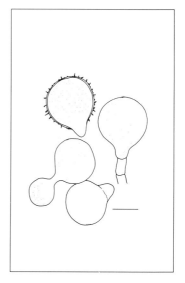

Bibliography:
Kwon-Chung, Bennett, 1992
O'Donnell, 1979

Figure 29.1 *Conidiobolus coronatus.*

100

Figure 29.2   *Conidiobolus coronatus.*
Potato glucose agar,
25°C, 7 days.

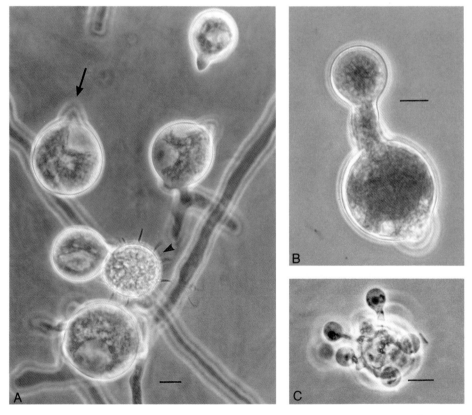

Figure 29.3   *Conidiobolus coronatus.* A, Free sporangiole with papilla↑;
villose sporangiole▲. B, Primary sporangiole producing a
secondary sporangiole. C, Primary sporangiole surrounded
by a crown of secondary sporangioles.

101

Cunninghamella   Matruchot, 1903

Pathogenicity: *Cunninghamella bertholletiae*, a fungus in the order Mucorales, is occasionally an agent of pulmonary or disseminated zygomycosis in the
severely debilitated patient.

Ecology: *Cunninghamella* species are soil saprobes mainly found in Mediterranean or subtropical climatic zones.

Colony appearance:
- very rapid growth;
- cottony texture;
- color white to grey on the surface; reverse pale.

Microscopic appearance:
- hyphae broad, aseptate or with very infrequent septa;
- sporangiophores branched, terminating in a vesicle;
- one-spored sporangioles formed on denticles on the vesicle surface.

Remarks: *Cunninghamella* is distinguished by its broad hyphae, aseptate or
nearly so, and its sporangiophores terminating in a vesicle supporting sporangioles containing a single sporangiospore. *C. bertholletiae* is the only pathogenic species; isolates from clinical sources differ from the very similar, nonpathogenic *Cunninghamella elegans* by their growth at 40°C.

Bibliography:
Domsch, Gams, Anderson, 1980
McGinnis, 1980
Scholer, Müller, Schipper, 1983
Weitzman, 1984

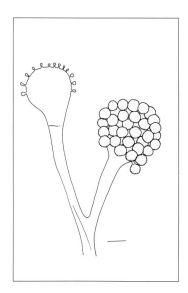

Figure 30.1   *Cunning-
hamella*
sp.

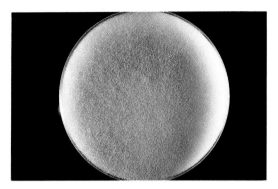

Figure 30.2 *Cunninghamella bertholletiae.* Potato glucose agar, 25°C, 7 days.

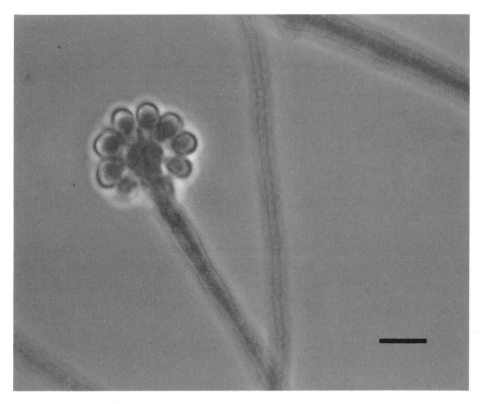

Figure 30.3 *Cunninghamella bertholletiae.* One-spored sporangioles developing from a vesicle formed at the tip of the sporangiophore.

103

Curvularia Boedijn, 1933

Pathogenicity: occasionally a cause of human infection, including ony-chomycosis, keratitis, sinusitis, mycetoma, pneumonia, endocarditis, cerebral abscess, and disseminated infection. A significant proportion of these cases are from immunocompetent patients. Mycetomas are most frequently encountered in animals.

Ecology: most species are facultative pathogens of tropical or subtropical plants, but a few are commonly isolated in temperate agricultural areas.

Colony appearance:
- rapid growth;
- wooly texture;
- color white becoming olive brown on the surface and the reverse.

Microscopic appearance:
- hyphae septate, brown;
- conidiophores brown, geniculate, simple or branched;
- poroconidia slightly but distinctly curved, brown, transversely multiseptate, with a central cell typically expanded and darker than the other cells.

Remarks: *Curvularia* is distinguished by its multicellular, somewhat curved conidia with a larger and darker central cell. Unlike *Bipolaris* and *Drechslera*, the conidia are septate from side wall to side wall, not distoseptate.

Bibliography:
de Hoog, 1983
Domsch, Gams, Anderson, 1980
Kwon-Chung, Bennett, 1992

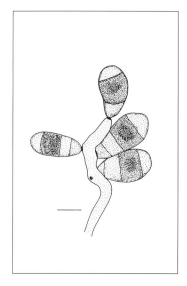

Figure 31.1 *Curvularia* sp.

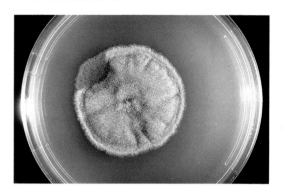

Figure 31.2 Potato glucose agar,
25°C, 7 days.

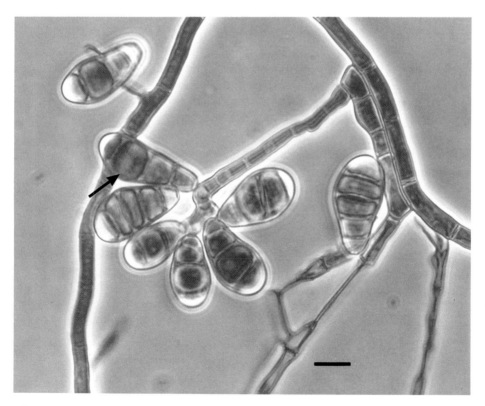

Figure 31.3 *Curvularia* sp. Curved poroconidia with larger and darker
central cell↑.

Drechslera Ito, 1930

Pathogenicity: *Drechslera biseptata*, recently isolated from a brain abscess in a patient apparently lacking any predisposing condition, is the sole species known to cause human or animal disease. *Drechslera* species previously reported as pathogenic are today considered members of the genera *Bipolaris* and *Exserohilum*.

Ecology: cosmopolitan, isolated from soil and plants. Some species are plant pathogens.

Colony appearance:
- rapid growth;
- texture velvety to wooly;
- color white becoming olive brown to black on the surface and on the reverse.

Microscopic appearance:
- hyphae septate, brown;
- conidiophores brown, simple or branched, geniculate;
- poroconidia brown, fusoid, distoseptate, without a protuberant hilum;
- germ tube developing perpendicularly to the long axis of the conidium.

Remarks: *Drechslera* is distinguished from *Exserohilum* by its conidia lacking protuberant hila. Unlike *Bipolaris*, it produces germ tubes from any cell of the conidium, not just the end cells, and these germ tubes tend to grow out perpendicularly to the conidial long axis. Isolates of *Drechslera* have a tendency to become sterile in laboratory cultivation. Sporulation can sometimes be stimulated by cultivating isolates on V-8 agar exposed to periodic ultraviolet light.

Bibliography:
de Hoog, 1983
Kwon-Chung, Bennett, 1992
McGinnis, Rinaldi, Winn, 1986

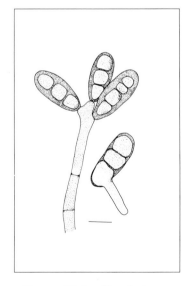

Figure 32.1   *Drechslera biseptata.*

106

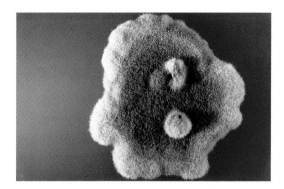

Figure 32.2   *Drechslera biseptata.*
Potato glucose agar,
25°C, 7 days.

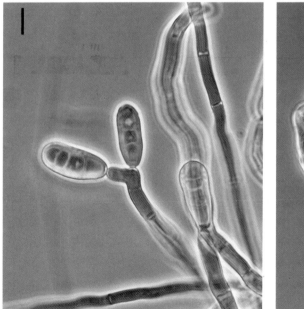
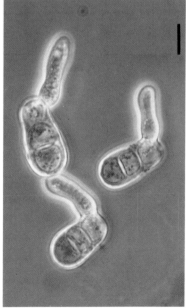

Figure 32.3   *Drechslera biseptata.* A, Geniculate conidiophore and conidia
with rounded base and hilar scar not or scarcely protuberant.
B, Germ tubes growing perpendicular to the long axis of the
conidium. (Courtesy of M. McGinnis).

Emmonsia

Ciferri et Montemartini, 1953

Pathogenicity: *Emmonsia parva* (= *Chrysosporium parvum*) is the etiologic agent of adiaspiromycosis, a usually asymptomatic pulmonary infection encountered in animals and more rarely in humans. The disseminated form of the infection is rarely seen in the immunocompromised host. *E. parva* var. *crescens* is the only type isolated from humans, while *E. parva* var. *parva* is often isolated from animals.

Ecology: cosmopolitan, soil saprobes. Isolated from numerous mammalian species, especially small rodents.

Colony appearance:
- moderately rapid growth;
- texture velvety;
- color white to chamois on the surface; reverse pale.

Microscopic appearance:
- hyphae septate, hyaline;
- conidiophores simple or sometimes branching at right angles;
- conidia (aleurioconidia) hyaline, unicellular, rather rounded, lightly roughened, usually solitary or in short chains of 2 to 3 cells.
- adiaspores formed at 37°C or 40°C on blood agar.

Remarks: the conidia of *E. parva*, unlike those of *Chrysosporium*, may inflate and become transformed into adiaspores when incubated at 37°C or 40°C. *E. parva* comprises two varieties: the variety *crescens* is distinguished from the variety *parva* by forming adiaspores at 37°C rather than 40°C. Further, the adiaspores of the variety *crescens* may attain diameters of 70 µm *in vitro* and 700 µm *in vivo*, while those of the variety *parva* do not exceed 25 µm *in vitro* and 40 µm *in vivo*. Unlike *Blastomyces dermatitidis*, *E. parva* does not convert to a yeast phase at 37°C, and unlike *Sporotrichum*, it does not produce large chlamydospores at 25°C.

Bibliography:
Carmichael, 1962
Kwon-Chung, Bennett, 1992
van Oorschot, 1980

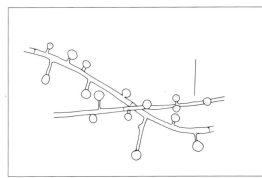

Figure 33.1   *Emmonsia parva.*

Figure 33.2 *Emmonsia parva* var. *crescens*. Potato glucose agar, 25°C, 7 days.

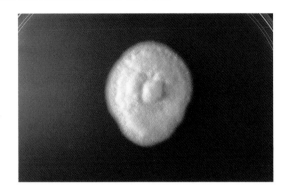

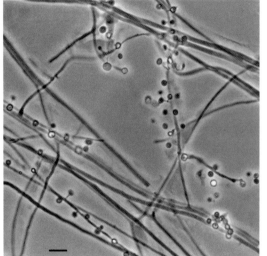

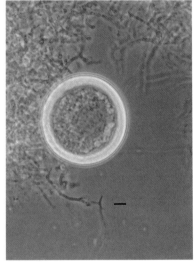

Figure 33.3 *Emmonsia parva* var. *crescens*. A, Conidia at 25°C. B, Adiaspores at 37°C on blood agar.

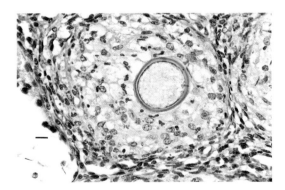

Figure 33.4 *Emmonsia parva* var. *parva*. Adiaspore in mouse tissue.

Epicoccum Link, 1815

Pathogenicity: no cases of infection have been reported in humans or animals.

Ecology: cosmopolitan, isolated from infected plants or from litter or soil.

Colony appearance:
- rapid growth;
- texture felty to wooly;
- color yellow, orange, red or brown on the surface; reverse deep brown with orange or brown pigment diffusing in the medium.

Microscopic appearance:
- hyphae septate, hyaline to brownish;
- conidiophores short, little differentiated from vegetative hyphae, grouped in compact clusters (sporodochia);
- conidia brown, muriform, rough-walled, more or less round.

Remarks: *Epicoccum* is distinguished by its yellow orange to brown colonies producing clumps of brown, muriform conidia. These clumps are sometimes visible as brown spots on the surface of the colony. Sporulation of initially nonsporulating isolates can be stimulated by subculturing on 2% agar.

Bibliography:
Domsch, Gams, Anderson, 1980
McGinnis, 1980

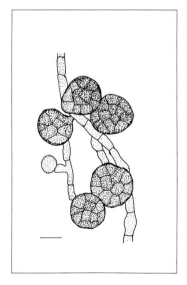

Figure 34.1 *Epicoccum* sp.

110

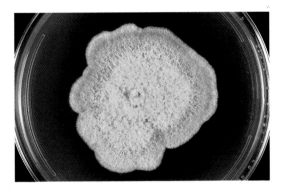

Figure 34.2   Potato glucose agar,
25°C, 7 days.

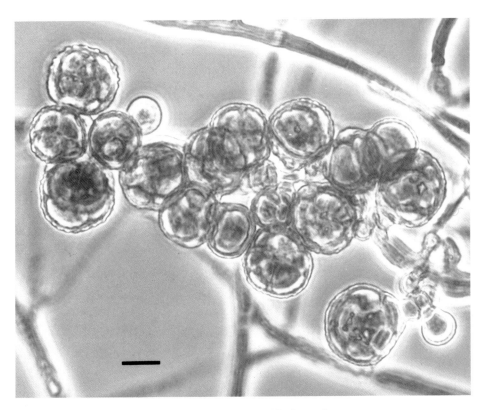

Figure 34.3   *Epicoccum* sp.   Muriform conidia in a clump.

Epidermophyton Sabouraud, 1907

Pathogenicity: *Epidermophyton floccosum* is a dermatophyte commonly responsible for cutaneous infections, particularly of the groin and of the feet.

Ecology: cosmopolitan, anthropophilic.

Colony appearance:
- slow growth;
- texture membranous becoming felty to powdery;
- color yellow to khaki on the surface; with reverse chamois to brown.

Microscopic appearance:
- macroconidia club-shaped, with thin, smooth walls, solitary or in groups;
- microconidia absent;
- chlamydospores formed in large numbers in mature colonies.

Remarks: *E. floccosum* is distinguished from other dermatophytes by its restricted, yellow to khaki colonies, its club-shaped macroconidia with thin, smooth walls, and its inability to form microconidia. Cultures rapidly manifest pleomorphism, in which white, atypical sectors soon arise on the colony surface. This phenomenon can be deterred by maintaining strains on Sabouraud glucose agar containing 3 to 5% sodium chloride.

Bibliography:
Kwon-Chung, Bennett, 1992
Rebell, Taplin, 1972
Weitzman, Kane, 1991

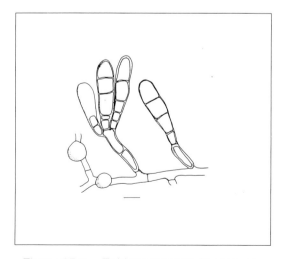

Figure 35.1 *Epidermophyton floccosum.*

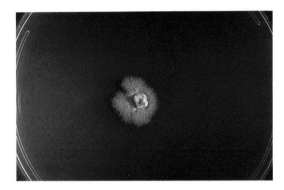

Figure 35.2   *Epidermophyton floccosum.*
Sabouraud glucose agar,
25°C, 7 days.

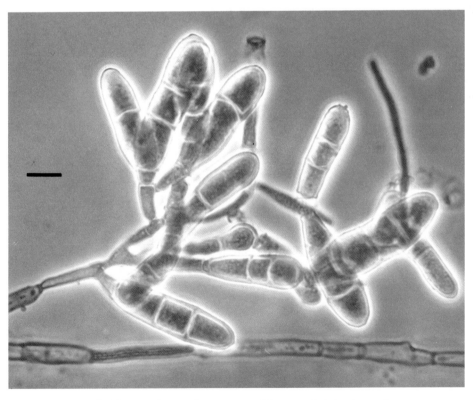

Figure 35.3   *Epidermophyton floccosum.*   Cluster of club-shaped
macroconidia.

113

Exophiala   Carmichael, 1966

Pathogenicity: occasionally a cause of mycetomas and of other subcutaneous phaeohyphomycoses. *Exophiala werneckii* is the etiologic agent of a superficial infection known as tinea nigra. *Exophiala* infections have also been reported from animals, especially fish.

Ecology: cosmopolitan, isolated from decaying wood, soil, and surfaces in contact with cool, fresh water. Occasional contaminants of feet and nails.

Colony appearance:
- slow growth;
- texture mucoid becoming velvety;
- color dark brown to black on the surface and on the reverse.

Microscopic appearance:
- hyphae septate, pale brown;
- annellides pigmented brown, cylindrical or slightly inflated, with a rather pointed tip; the entire structure often little differentiated from the vegetative hyphae;
- conidia hyaline or pale brown, oval to cylindrical, unicellular or bicellular, accumulating at the tip of the annellides or sliming down its length;
- yeast cells unicellular or bicellular, mostly present at the beginning of colony formation.

Remarks: *Exophiala jeanselmei* is the principal species of medical importance. It differs from *Wangiella dermatitidis* in not growing at 40°C and in assimilating potassium nitrate as a sole nitrogen source. In contrast to *Phialophora*, in which phialides terminate in a collarette, the conidiogenous cells of *Exophiala* are little differentiated from vegetative hyphae and are rather pointed at the tip. *Exophiala spinifera* is distinguished from *E. jeanselmei* by its spine-like annellides, produced on conidiophores several cells long. *E. werneckii* typically produces bicellular yeasts terminating in an annellide at one end.

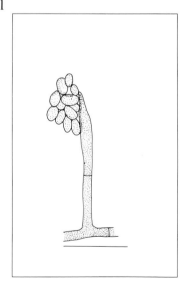

Figure 36.1   *Exophiala jeanselmei.*

114

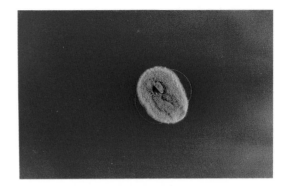

Figure 36.2 *Exophiala jeanselmei.*
Potato glucose agar,
25°C, 7 days.

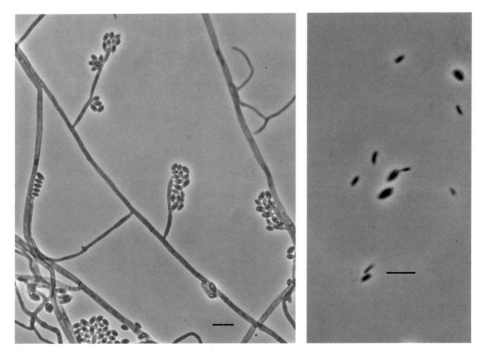

Figure 36.3 *Exophiala jeanselmei.* A, Annellides and conidia. B, Yeast cells.

115

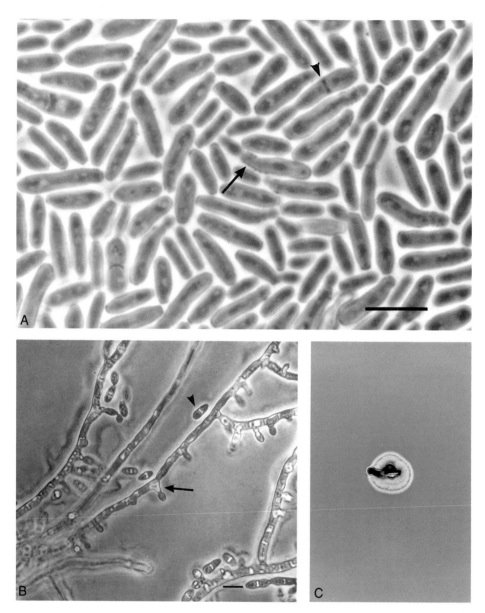

Figure 36.4   *Exophiala werneckii*. A, Bicellular yeasts▲ with a rugose process[↑]
(annellidic neck) at one end. B, Annellide[↑], little differentiated
and intercalated in an otherwise unspecialized hypha; bicellular
conidium▲. C, Sabouraud glucose agar, 25°C, 7 days.

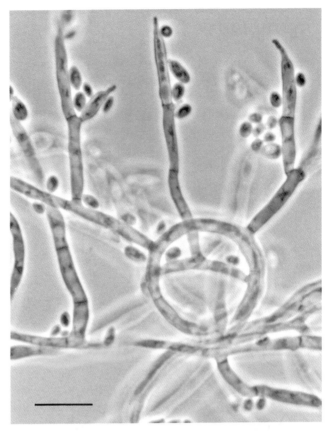

Figure 36.5   *Exophiala spinifera.* Spine-like
annellides produced on
conidiophores several cells long.

Bibliography:
Dixon, Polak-Wyss, 1990
de Hoog, 1983
Kwon-Chung, 1992
McGinnis, 1980

Exserohilum

Leonard et Suggs, 1974

Pathogenicity: some cases of subcutaneous or deep phaeohyphomycosis have been reported in humans and animals.

Ecology: cosmopolitan, facultative plant pathogens also occasionally isolated from soil.

Colony appearance:
- moderately rapid growth;
- texture velvety;
- color dark olive to black on the surface and reverse.

Microscopic appearance:
- hyphae septate, pale brown;
- conidiophores brown, geniculate at the apex;
- poroconidia cylindrical to ellipsoidal, multicellular, distoseptate, with a protuberant hilum at the base;
- germ tubes developing in the direction of the conidial long axis or on the side.

Remarks: *Exserohilum* is distinguished from *Bipolaris* and *Drechslera* by their conidia with a protuberant hilum. In many species, the end cells of the conidia are delimited by strongly darkened septa.

Bibliography:
Kwon-Chung, Bennett, 1992
McGinnis, Rinaldi, Winn, 1986

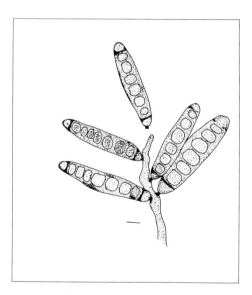

Figure 37.1   *Exserohilum* sp.

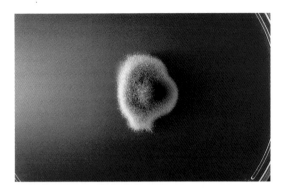

Figure 37.2 *Exserohilum mcginnisii*.
Potato glucose agar,
25°C, 7 days.

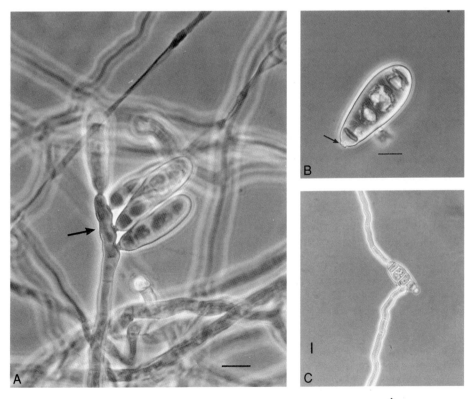

Figure 37.3 *Exserohilum mcginnisii*. A, Geniculate conidiophore$^\uparrow$.
B, Poroconidium with protuberant hilum$^\uparrow$ and darker
septa at the ends. C, Conidium with germ tubes.
(Courtesy of M. McGinnis).

119

Fonsecaea   Negroni, 1936

Pathogenicity: *Fonsecaea* species are agents of chromoblastomycosis, a chronic subcutaneous infection characterized by verrucous lesions and the formation of brown, sclerotic fission cells ("copper pennies") in tissue. It is often confined to a single limb.

Ecology: isolated from soil and from decomposing plant materials. Most cases of infection come from tropical and subtropical regions.

Colony appearance:
- slow growth;
- texture downy;
- color brownish black, olive brown, grey black or jet black on the surface and the reverse.

Microscopic appearance:
- hyphae septate, brown;
- conidiophores cylindrical, slightly inflated at the tip;
- blastoconidia unicellular, ellipsoid to round, formed sympodially in successive ranks;
- conidiophores and conidia in arrangements of the *Rhinocladiella* and *Cladosporium* types often present; phialides of the *Phialophora* type with prominent collarettes rarely present.

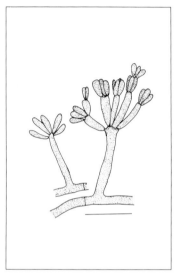

Figure 38.1 *Fonsecaea pedrosoi.*

Remarks: *Fonsecaea* species are polymorphous fungi which produce several types of conidial structures. The most characteristic is composed of a conidiophore with successive ranks of conidia at its apex. Arrangements of the *Rhinocladiella* and *Cladosporium* types are often present, while the *Phialophora* form is only encountered sporadically. The genus *Fonsecaea* comprises two species, *F. pedrosoi* and *F. compacta*. *F. compacta* is by far the rarer of the two and is distinguished by conidia more round than ellipsoid, with broad attachment points, and a conidiogenous structure more compact overall in construction.

Bibliography:
Kwon-Chung, 1992
McGinnis, 1980;
Rippon, 1988

Figure 38.2 *Fonsecaea pedrosoi.* Potato glucose agar, 25°C, 7 days.

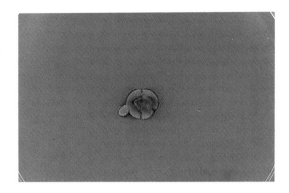

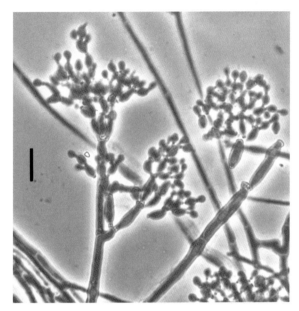
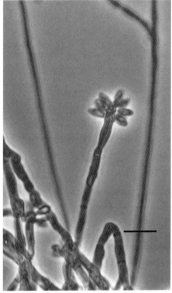

Figure 38.3 *Fonsecaea pedrosoi.* A, Conidia in successive ranks. B, Conidial structure of the *Rhinocladiella* type.

Figure 38.4 *Fonsecaea compacta.* Conidia oval to round with broad attachment points↑.

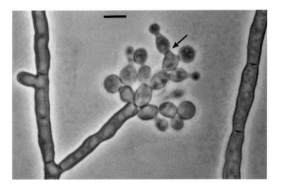

Fusarium Link, 1809

Pathogenicity: occasionally a cause of keratitis, endophthalmitis, ony-chomycosis or mycetoma. Also a cause of disseminated infection in the immunocompromised patient and of peritonitis in the ambulatory dialysis patient.

Ecology: cosmopolitan, frequently isolated from soil. Certain species are important plant pathogens; others produce toxins in grains or stored animal feed.

Colony appearance:
- rapid growth;
- texture usually wooly, sometimes mucoid;
- color white, yellow, pink, purple, or pale brown on the surface; reverse pale, red, violet, brown, or sometimes blue.

Microscopic appearance:
- hyphae septate, hyaline;
- phialides long or short, cylindrical, simple or branched, with a scarcely discernible collarette at the apex;
- microconidia unicellular, sometimes bicellular, hyaline, ovoid to ellipsoid, in slimy heads or in chains;
- macroconidia curved, multicellular, with a foot cell at the base;
- chlamydospores sometimes present.

Remarks: typically *Fusarium* is distinguished from *Acremonium* by its curved, multicellular macroconidia. Nonetheless, some species produce few or no macroconidia on media routinely used in medical mycology; in comparison to *Acremonium*, their colonies are wooly and develop more rapidly, attaining a diameter of 3 cm or more in 7 days. *Cylindrocarpon* is distinguished from *Fusarium* by its straight to curved macroconidia lacking a foot cell.

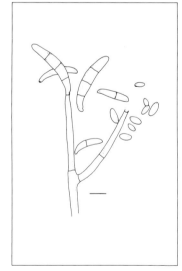

Bibliography:
Booth, 1971
Domsch, Gams, Anderson, 1980
Guarro, Gene, 1992
Kwon-Chung, Bennett, 1992
Nelson, Toussoun, Marasas, 1983

Figure 39.1 *Fusarium sp.*

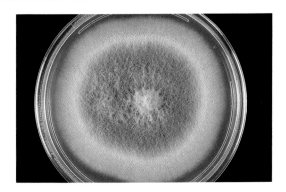

Figure 39.2   Potato glucose agar,
25°C, 7 days.

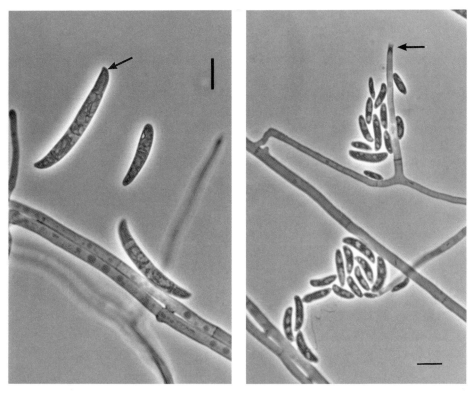

Figure 39.3   *Fusarium* sp. A, Macroconidia with foot cell[↑]. B, Phialide with
collarette[↑].

Geotrichum
Link, 1809

Pathogenicity: whether concerning cutaneous or deep infections, most of the cases reported to date lack proper documentation or are based on unreliable identifications.

Ecology: cosmopolitan saprobes, isolated from soil and plants and frequently from milk and milk products. *Geotrichum candidum* is considered part of the normal microbiota of humans; it is frequently isolated from sputum samples, faeces, urine, and vaginal secretions.

Colony appearance:
- rapid growth;
- texture creamy becoming powdery to waxy;
- color white on surface and reverse.

Microscopic appearance:
- hyphae septate, hyaline;
- conidiophores absent;
- arthroconidia rectangular, not alternating, liberated by the fission of double walls;
- blastoconidia (i.e., budding yeast cells) absent.

Remarks: *G. candidum* is distinguished from *Trichosporon* by not producing urease; it differs from *Blastoschizomyces capitatus* by its assimilation of D-xylose. In general, *Geotrichum* is distinguished from the majority of arthroconidial filamentous fungi by its creamy or waxy, rather than wooly colonies. More specifically, it differs from *Arthrographis* by its absence of conidiophores and from *Malbranchea* and *Coccidioides* by the absence of disjunctors between the arthroconidia.

Bibliography:
Kwon-Chung, Bennett, 1992
McGinnis, 1980
de Hoog, Smith, Guého, 1986

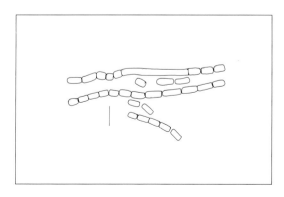

Figure 40.1   *Geotrichum* sp.

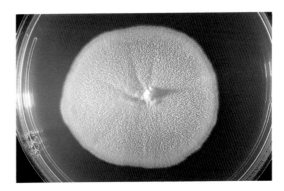

Figure 40.2 *Geotrichum candidum.*
Potato glucose agar,
25°C, 7 days.

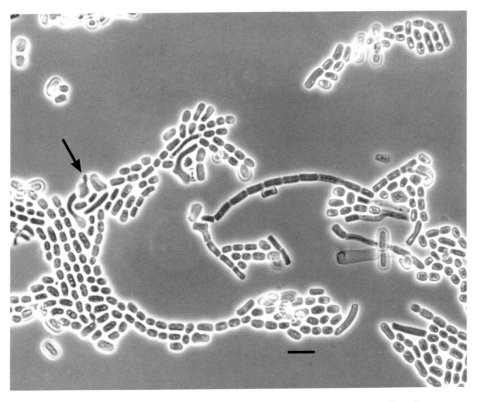

Figure 40.3 *Geotrichum candidum.* Rectangular arthroconidia, closely
apposed; beginning of germination↑.

Gliocladium

Corda, 1840

Pathogenicity: no case of infection has been recorded in humans or animals.

Ecology: cosmopolitan, saprobes frequently isolated from soil and decaying plant materials.

Colony appearance:
- rapid growth;
- texture wooly;
- color white, pink or green on the surface; reverse pale or yellow.

Microscopic appearance:
- hyphae septate, hyaline;
- conidiophores branched in the upper portions;
- phialides in brush-like clusters;
- conidia unicellular, slimy, smooth-walled, accumulating in a viscous mass at the tips of the phialides.

Remarks: *Gliocladium* is distinguished by its branching conidiophores supporting phialides in brush-like (penicillate) clusters, with masses of viscous conidia at the apices.

Bibliography:
Domsch, Gams, Anderson, 1980
McGinnis, 1980

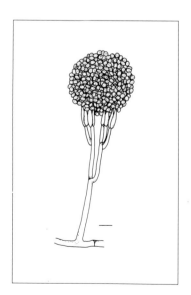

Figure 41.1 *Gliocladium* sp.

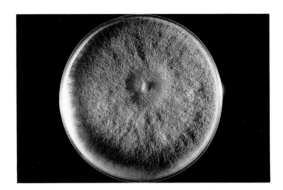

Figure 41.2   Potato glucose agar,
25°C, 7 days.

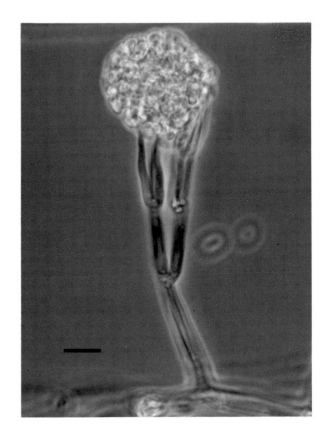

Figure 41.3   *Gliocladium* sp. Mass of conidia at
the apex of phialides grouped in
a brush-like cluster.

Helminthosporium Link, 1809: Fries (nom. cons.)

Pathogenicity: no case of infection has reliably been linked to *Helminthosporium* in humans or animals. Some cases reported in the past were caused by fungi now identified as *Exserohilum* or *Bipolaris* species.

Ecology: isolated from plants, where they sometimes play a role as pathogens.

Colony appearance:
- rapid growth;
- texture downy to wooly;
- color olive brown to black on surface and reverse.

Microscopic appearance:
- hyphae septate, brown;
- conidiophores brown, with parallel walls, and with determinate growth, that is, ceasing to elongate once the first conidium is formed;
- poroconidia obclavate, transversely multiseptate, formed along the perimeter of the conidiophore.

Remarks: *Helminthosporium* is distinguished from *Bipolaris*, *Drechslera* and *Exserohilum* by its stiffly erect rather than geniculate conidiophores and by the obclavate shape (larger at the base) of its conidia.

Bibliography:
McGinnis, 1980
McGinnis, Rinaldi, Winn, 1986

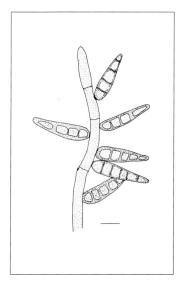

Figure 42.1   *Helmintho-
sporium*
sp.

128

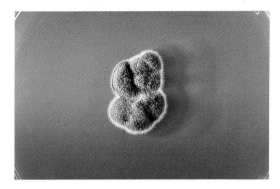

Figure 42.2   Potato glucose agar,
25°C, 7 days.

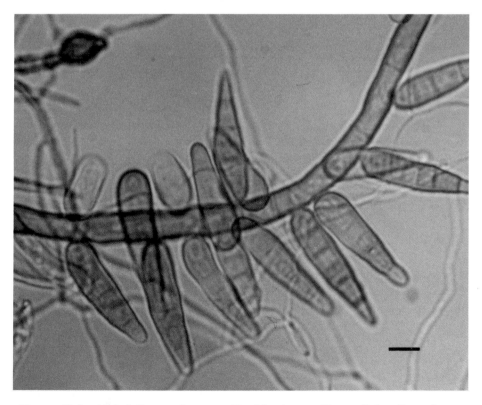

Figure 42.3   *Helminthosporium* sp. Conidiophore with parallel walls and
obclavate poroconidia.

Histoplasma capsulatum   Darling, 1906

Pathogenicity: *Histoplasma capsulatum* is the etiologic agent of histoplasmosis, an infection most often presenting in a benign pulmonary form, but occasionally progressing to a life- threatening, disseminated form particularly affecting the reticuloendothelial system.

Ecology: mostly isolated from nitrogen-rich soils contaminated by excrement of birds or bats. Despite its world-wide distribution, the organism is often encountered in tropical or subtropical regions, as well as in several large river basins in temperate regions. The valleys of the Mississippi and the Ohio rivers in the United States are known for their high degree of endemicity.

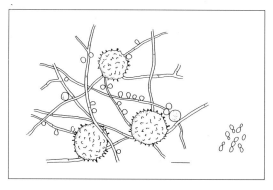

Figure 43.1   *Histoplasma capsulatum.* Filamentous form and yeast form.

DIMORPHIC FUNGUS

Colony appearance:

at 25°C:

- slow growth;
- texture wooly to granular;
- color white becoming brownish on the surface and yellowish on the reverse.

at 37°C, on rich medium:

- slow growth;
- texture creamy;
- color cream on surface and reverse.

Microscopic appearance:

at 25°C:

- hyphae septate, hyaline;
- macroconidia (macroaleurioconidia) unicellular, hyaline, thick-walled, smooth or warty;
- microconidia (microaleurioconidia) unicellular, hyaline, with wall smooth or rough.

at 37°C, on rich medium or in infected tissues:

- budding yeasts.

Remarks: *Histoplasma capsulatum* is a pathogenic fungus which should only be manipulated in culture in a biological safety cabinet in a containment laboratory. It is distinguished from *Chrysosporium* by its production of tuberculate macroconidia, and from *Sepedonium* by the production of microaleurioconidia. Additionally, it converts to a yeast phase at 37°C on rich media. The transition from the filamentous phase to the yeast phase may sometimes require several weeks of incubation. To speed the identification process and to reduce the risk of laboratory-acquired infection, most mycology laboratories today prefer to identify the organism by specific exoantigen testing or nucleic acid hybridization studies. *H. capsulatum* encompasses two varieties: the variety *capsulatum*, the more widespread of the two, which produces small yeasts 2-4 μm in length, and the variety *duboisii*, present primarily in Africa, which characteristically produces much larger yeasts measuring 12-15 μm.

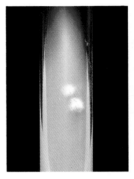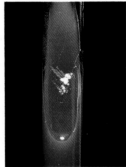

Bibliography:
Kwon-Chung, Bennett, 1992
McGinnis, 1980
Rippon, 1988

Figure 43.2   A, Filamentous form on Sabouraud glucose agar, 25°C, 7 days. B, Yeast form on blood agar, 37°C, 7 days.

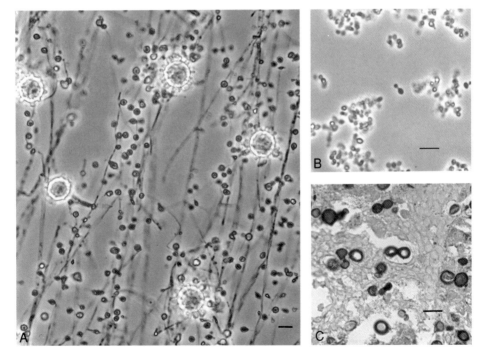

Figure 43.3   *Histoplasma capsulatum* var. *capsulatum*. A, Tuberculate macroconidia and microconidia. B, Yeasts. C, *Histoplasma capsulatum* var. *duboisii*. Yeasts in tissue.

Hormographiella

Guarro et Gené, gen. nov. 1992

Pathogenicity: no cases of infection have been recorded in humans or animals.

Ecology: cosmopolitan, isolated from dung, air, and human skin.

Colony appearance:
- rapid growth;
- texture downy to floccose;
- color white to cream on the surface and the reverse, sometimes becoming brownish with age.

Microscopic appearance:
- hyphae septate, hyaline;
- conidiophores erect, simple or branched, septate, producing conidiogenous hyphae which fragment to form arthroconidia;
- arthroconidia in short chains, without disjunctor cells, hyaline, cylindrical, non-septate, produced in whorls or tufts at the apex of conidiophores;
- brown sclerotia sometimes present in older cultures.

Remarks: *Hormographiella* is characterized by its broad, erect conidiophores with whorls or tufts of arthroconidia at the apex, and by its growth more rapid at 37°C than at 25°C.

Bibliography:
Guarro, Gené, de Vroey, Guého, 1992

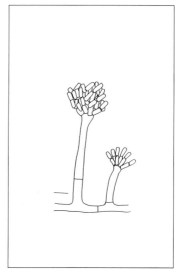

Figure 44.1   *Hormo-graphiella* sp.

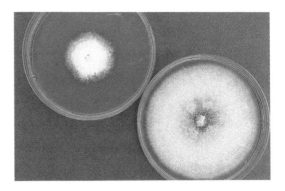

Figure 44.2   Potato glucose agar, 25°C
and 37°C, 7 days.

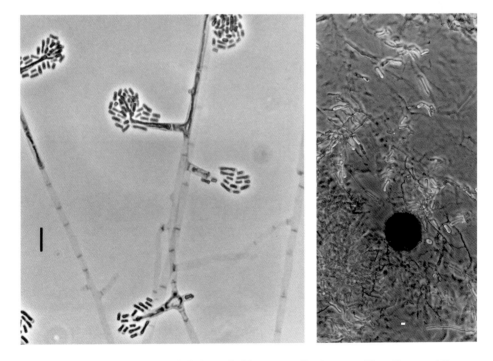

Figure 44.3   *Hormographiella* sp. A, Erect condiophores with arthroconidia
in whorls. B, Dark sclerotium.

133

Lecythophora   Nannfeldt, 1934

Pathogenicity: only two cases of endocarditis, one of peritonitis and one gluteal abscess have been reported from humans.

Ecology: cosmopolitan, occasionally isolated from decaying plant material and from soil.

Colony appearance:
- moderately rapid growth;
- texture slimy becoming lightly downy at the center of the colony;
- color pale pink to salmon on the surface and on the reverse, sometimes becoming pale to deep brown.

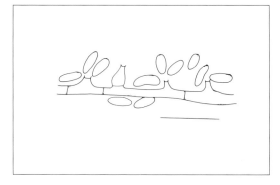

Figure 45.1   *Lecythophora hoffmannii.*

Microscopic appearance:
- hyphae septate, hyaline;
- phialides mostly not septate at the base (adelophialides), short, cylindrical or conical, often solitary, sometimes grouped on short lateral filaments;
- phialides with septate bases occasionally present;
- conidia hyaline, ellipsoidal to cylindrical, sometimes slightly curved, and sometimes giving rise to secondary conidia;
- brown chlamydospores sometimes present.

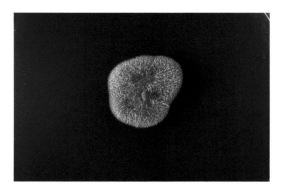

Figure 45.2   *Lecythophora hoffmannii.*
Potato glucose agar,
25°C, 7 days.

Remarks: *Lecythophora* species, formerly regarded as members of the genus *Phialophora*, are distinguished by their phialides which are not septate at the base (adelophialides). Unlike *Lecythophora hoffmanii*, which has pink colonies, *Lecythophora mutabilis* produces numerous brown chlamydospores which give mature colonies a brown color. *Lecythophora lignicola* also produces colonies which become brown, but in this case the pigment develops in the hyphae alone, since chlamydospores are absent.

Bibliography:
Gams, McGinnis, 1983
de Hoog, 1983
Kwon-Chung, Bennett, 1992

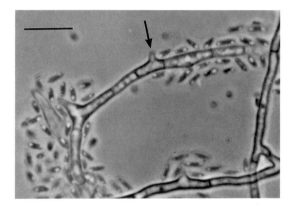

Figure 45.3   *Lecythophora hoffmannii.*
Adelophialide[↑] intercalated
in a hypha.

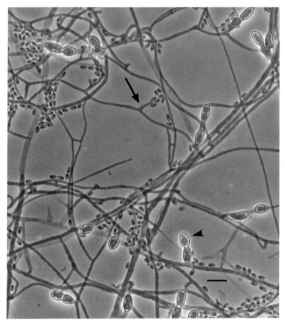
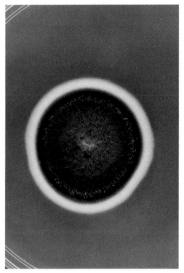

Figure 45.4   *Lecythophora mutabilis.* A, Adelophialide[↑] and
chlamydospore[▲]. B, Potato glucose agar, 25°C, 7 days.

Madurella Brumpt, 1905

Pathogenicity: *Madurella* is among the fungi responsible for black grain mycetoma.

Ecology: saprobes with distribution restricted to certain tropical and subtropical areas in Africa, India, and South America.

Colony appearance:
- slow growth;
- texture glabrous to wooly;
- color white, yellow-brown, olive brown to dark grey on the surface; reverse dark brown, sometimes with the production of a brown diffusible pigment.

Microscopic appearance:
- hyphae septate, sometimes toruloid, normally sterile;
- chlamydospores or sclerotia sometimes present;
- phialides with vase shaped collarettes occasionally produced by *Madurella mycetomatis* on weak media.

Remarks: isolates of *Madurella* are normally sterile, and are difficult to distinguish from other sterile dematiaceous fungi. Isolation from a mycetoma with black grains is the most distinctive identification character. *Madurella grisea* differs from M. *mycetomatis* by growing poorly or not at all at 37°C and by not assimilating sucrose.

Bibliography:
Kwon-Chung, Bennett, 1992
McGinnis, 1980
Rippon, 1988

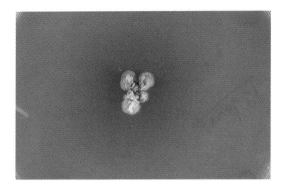

Figure 46.1   *Madurella mycetomatis.*
Potato glucose agar,
25°C, 7 days.

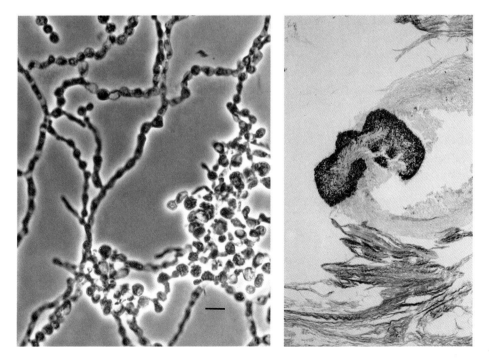

Figure 46.2   *Madurella mycetomatis.* A, Toruloid hyphae and
chlamydospores. B, Black grain in bone tissue.

Malbranchea

Saccardo, 1882

Pathogenicity: no cases of infection have been substantiated in humans or animals.

Ecology: cosmopolitan, isolated from soil, animal dung, and decaying plant materials.

Colony appearance:
- moderately rapid growth;
- texture powdery to wooly;
- color white, orange, beige, or sometimes brown.

Microscopic appearance:
- hyphae septate, hyaline;
- conidiophores absent;
- arthroconidia unicellular, rectangular, of the same diameter as the hyphae from which they are formed, alternating with empty cells (disjunctors); separated arthroconidia bear an annular frill which is a remnant of the wall of the disjunctor.

Remarks: *Malbranchea* produces alternate arthroconidia which, at the time they are formed, are of the same width as the hyphae. Once liberated following the lysis of the disjunctors, these arthroconidia, much like those of *Coccidioides immitis*, possess an annular frill. Given close resemblance of *Malbranchea* to *Coccidioides*, it is preferable to manipulate them in a biological safety cabinet until their identification is completed. They are best differentiated from *Coccidioides* by their negative reactions in the specific exoantigen or nucleic acid probe tests for the identification of this pathogen.

Bibliography:
McGinnis, 1980
Sigler, Carmichael, 1976

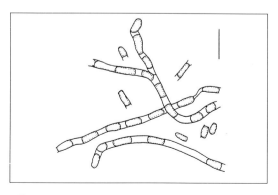

Figure 47.1   *Malbranchea* sp.

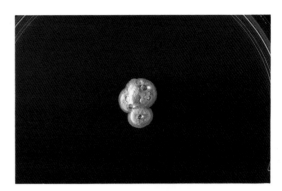

Figure 47.2 *Malbranchea* sp.
Potato glucose agar,
25°C, 7 days.

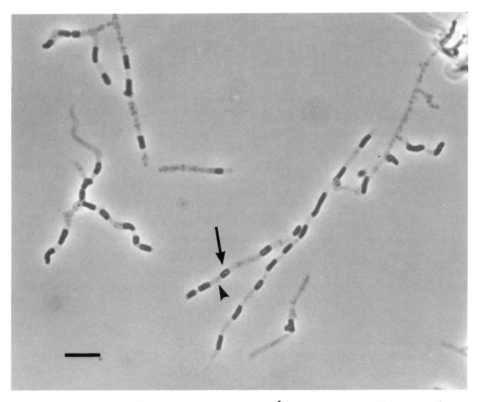

Figure 47.3   *Malbranchea* sp. Arthroconidia↑ alternating with disjunctors▲.

Microsporum Gruby, 1843

Pathogenicity: the genus *Microsporum* includes some 17 species, of which 5 are primarily isolated from humans and 7 primarily from animals. *Microsporum* infects the skin and the hair, but seldom infects nails.

Ecology: includes anthropophilic, zoophilic and geophilic species. Some are cosmopolitan while others have geographically restricted distributions.

Colony appearance:
* growth slow to rapid;
* texture glabrous, downy, or wooly;
* color white, beige, cinnamon, yellow or rusty on the surface; reverse pale, yellow, red, brown, or red-brown.

Microscopic appearance:
* hyphae septate;
* conidiophores scarcely or not differentiated from vegetative hyphae;
* microconidia (microaleurioconidia) unicellular, ovoid to club- shaped, solitary;
* macroconidia (macroaleurioconidia) fusiform, with a thick or thin, echinulate wall, solitary, containing 2 to 15 cells;
* some species are typically sterile but may sometimes form macroconidia on suitable media.

Remarks: from a taxonomic point of view, *Microsporum* is distinguished from *Trichophyton* and *Epidermophyton* by its fusiform macroconidia with rough to echinulate walls. In practice, the identification of many species rests primarily on the appearance of the macroconidia, since the microconidia are not sufficiently distinctive to be useful for this purpose. Some species, however, produce few or no macroconidia. The production of macroconidia can sometimes be stimulated by cultivating isolates on lactritmel agar, on autoclaved rice grains, on potato glucose agar or on Sabouraud glucose agar containing 3 to 5% sodium chloride. In the absence of conidia, the colony appearance and certain physiological tests are used in identification.

Bibliography:
Kwon-Chung, Bennett, 1992
Rebell, Taplin, 1970
Rippon, 1988
Vanbreuseghem, 1978
Weitzman, Kane, 1991

Table III. *Microsporum*: characteristics of selected species.

Species	Colony		Macroconidia	Microconidia	Hair perforation	Remarks
	Growth	Texture	Color (surface/reverse)				

Species	Growth	Texture	Color (surface/reverse)	Macroconidia	Microconidia	Hair perforation	Remarks
M. audouinii	moderately rapid	felt-like, downy	whitish / salmon	fusoid, deformed, very rare	absent or numerous	negative	poor growth on rice grains
M. canis	rapid	downy, woolly	white, yellowish / orange	fusoid, apex recurved, numerous	moderately numerous	positive	good growth on rice grains
M. cookei	moderately rapid	downy, powdery	white, yellowish / dark red	fusoid, numerous	numerous	positive	
M. ferrugineum	slow	glabrous	rusty to white / rusty, pale	absent	absent	negative	"bamboo" hyphae
M. gallinae	moderately rapid	downy	white, pinkish / red, diffusible	club-shaped, rare or numerous	rare or numerous	negative	
M. gypseum	rapid	powdery	beige / brown, yellowish	fusoid, symmetrical, numerous	moderately numerous	positive	
M. nanum	moderately rapid	powdery	white, yellowish / red brown	ovoid, 2-celled, numerous	moderately numerous	positive	avoid confusing with *Trichothecium*
M. persicolor	rapid	powdery	yellowish, pinkish / red brown	fusoid, club-shaped, sometimes present	numerous	positive	poor growth at 37°C

141

Microsporum audouinii Gruby, 1843

Pathogenicity: principally isolated from tinea infection of the scalp and of the glabrous skin in prepubescent children. Infected areas of the scalp and plucked hairs are fluorescent when examined under a Wood's light.

Ecology: an anthropophilic dermatophyte, cosmopolitan, extirpated in much of the world and now mainly present in Africa, Rumania and Haiti; it is rarely isolated in North America and Europe, mostly from migrants and travellers.

Colony appearance:
- moderately rapid growth;
- texture felty to downy;
- color greyish white to beige on the surface; reverse salmon or pale.

Microscopic appearance:
- hyphae septate, sometimes pectinate or with racquet cells;
- chlamydospores often present, terminal or intercalary;
- microconidia rare, club-shaped;
- macroconidia very rare, essentially spindle shaped but usually deformed, with wall at least partly echinulate.

Physiological tests:
- culture on autoclaved rice grains: little growth, brownish pigment
- hair perforation: negative
- growth factor requirements: none
- BCP-milk solids-glucose: alkalinization

Remarks: *M. audouinii* is recognized by its felty whitish colonies, with pinkish salmon reverse particularly evident on potato glucose agar. It usually produces terminal or intercalary chlamydospores. Unlike *Microsporum canis*, it grows poorly on autoclaved rice grains and produces an alkaline reaction on BCP- milk solids-glucose medium.

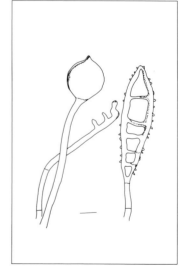

Figure 48.1   *Microsporum audouinii.*

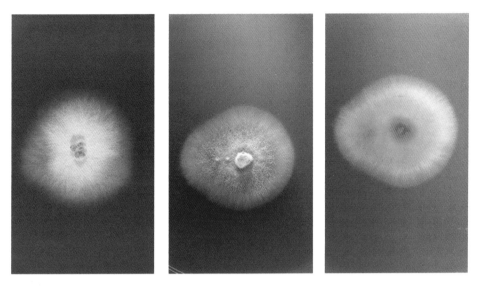

Figure 48.2   A, Sabouraud glucose agar, 25°C, 7 days. B, Potato glucose agar, 25°C, 7 days. (surface/reverse).

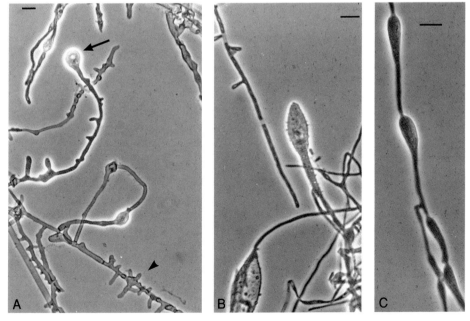

Figure 48.3   *Microsporum audouinii.* A, Terminal chlamydospore [↑] and pectinate hypha▲. B, Deformed, rough-walled macroconidium along with microconidia. C, Racquet hyphae.

Microsporum canis

Bodin, 1902

Pathogenicity: a frequent cause of tinea of the scalp and of the glabrous skin in humans. It is also often a cause of infection in animals. Infected areas of the scalp and plucked hairs are fluorescent when examined under a Wood's lamp.

Ecology: a cosmopolitan zoophilic dermatophyte, frequently isolated from cats and dogs.

Colony appearance:
- rapid growth;
- texture downy to wooly;
- color white to yellowish on the surface; reverse yellow to yellow orange, sometimes pale.

Microscopic appearance:
- microconidia club-shaped, infrequent;
- macroconidia numerous, fusoid, somewhat recurved at the apex, with a thick and echinulate cell wall, containing up to 15 cells.

Physiological tests:
- culture on autoclaved rice grains: good growth, white mycelium, yellow pigment
- hair perforation: positive
- growth factor requirements: none
- BCP-milk solids-glucose: no change of pH

Remarks: the colonies of *M. canis* are typically white to yellowish with a deep yellow reverse; they produce numerous fusoid macroconidia with thick and echinulate walls. Certain isolates are scarcely pigmented and/or sterile on Sabouraud glucose agar; the production of yellow pigment and macroconidia can be stimulated by cultivating isolates on lactritmel agar, on autoclaved rice grains or potato glucose agar.

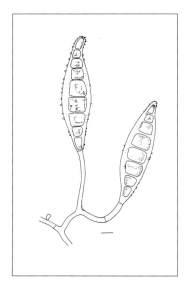

Figure 49.1   *Microsporum canis.*

144

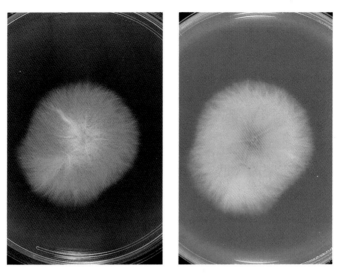

Figure 49.2   Sabouraud glucose agar, 25°C,
7 days (surface/reverse).

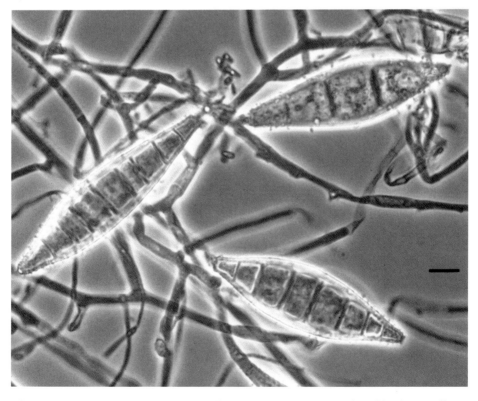

Figure 49.3   *Microsporum canis*. Fusoid macroconidia with echinulate wall.

145

Microsporum cookei Ajello, 1959

Pathogenicity: doubtful in both humans and animals.

Ecology: a cosmopolitan geophilic dermatophyte, occasionally isolated from cats, dogs and rodents.

Colony appearance:
- moderately rapid growth;
- texture downy becoming powdery;
- color white to yellow, sometimes becoming red brown or dark brown on the surface; reverse often dark red.

Microscopic appearance:
- microconidia ovoid, numerous;
- macroconidia fusoid, thick-walled, numerous.

Physiological tests:
- hair perforation: positive

Remarks: *M. cookei*, unlike *M. gypseum*, produces colonies with a red purple reverse and thick walled macroconidia.

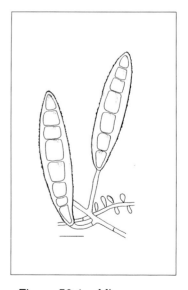

Figure 50.1   *Microsporum cookei.*

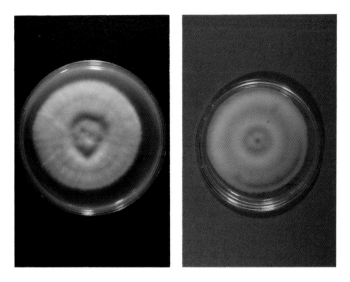

Figure 50.2   Potato glucose agar, 25°C,
14 days (surface/reverse).

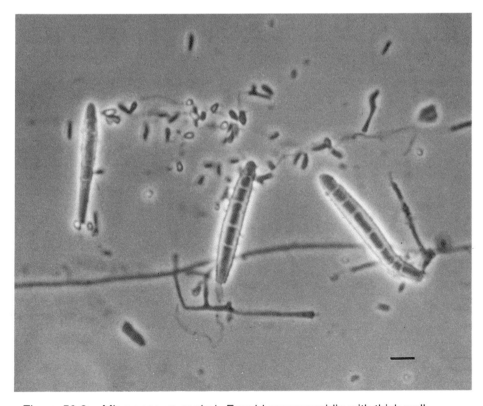

Figure 50.3   *Microsporum cookei*. Fusoid macroconidia with thick wall.

147

Microsporum ferrugineum Ota, 1921

Pathogenicity: frequent cause of tinea of the scalp in juveniles in certain endemic zones. No cases of infection have been reported in animals.

Ecology: an anthropophilic dermatophyte mostly encountered in Africa, east Asia, and eastern Europe.

Colony appearance:
- growth very slow to slow;
- texture glabrous to downy;
- color yellow, rusty or white on the surface; reverse rusty or scarcely pigmented.

Microscopic appearance:
- hyphae deformed or straight, with prominent "bamboo" septa;
- microconidia typically absent;
- macroconidia typically absent.

Physiological tests:
- hair perforation: negative
- urease: normally positive
- growth factor requirements: none
- Lowenstein-Jensen: pale yellow colonies.

Remarks: Typically, *M. ferrugineum* is a sterile dermatophyte which produces hyphae with a bamboo-like appearance. Those isolates which produce rusty yellow colonies can be distinguished from *Trichophyton soudanense* colonies by their pale yellow rather than brownish black color on Lowenstein-Jensen medium and by their positive urease test. In the laboratory, they have a tendency to become pleomorphic, soon becoming downy and white.

Bibliography:
Weitzman, Rosenthal, 1984

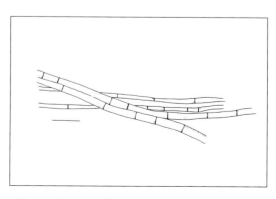

Figure 51.1 *Microsporum ferrugineum.*

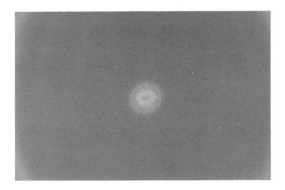

Figure 51.2   Sabouraud glucose agar,
25°C, 7 days.

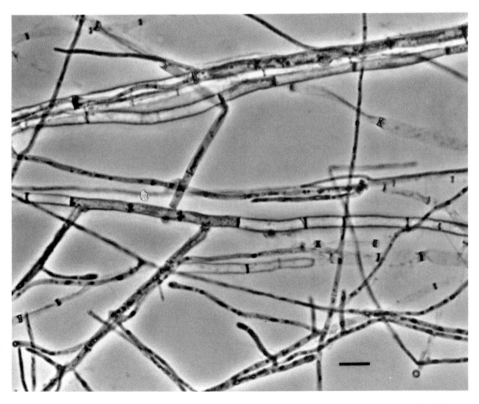

Figure 51.3   *Microsporum ferrugineum.* Hyphae with prominent "bamboo"
septa.

Microsporum gallinae

(Megnin) Grigorakis, 1929

Pathogenicity: seldom isolated from humans. A common cause of dermal infection in fowl, especially chickens and turkeys.

Ecology: cosmopolitan zoophilic dermatophyte, principally associated with fowl.

Colony appearance:
- moderately rapid growth;
- texture downy;
- color white to pink on the surface; reverse with deep red pigment diffusing into the medium.

Microscopic appearance:
- microconidia rare or numerous, ovoid to pyriform;
- macroconidia rare or numerous, club-shaped, often curved or more narrow at the apex, with a smooth or echinulate cell wall, containing 2 to 10 cells.

Physiological tests:
- hair perforation: negative
- growth factor requirements: none

Remarks: *M. gallinae* is distinguished by its roseate colonies which produce a vivid red diffusing pigment. Unlike *Trichophyton megninii*, *M. gallinae* does not have a requirement for histidine. It should be distinguished from *Myxotrichum deflexum*, a fungus which produces a red diffusing pigment but which, unlike *M. gallinae*, produces no conidia and instead, after 2 to 3 weeks of cultivation, forms clusters of stiff black hyphae ornamented with recurved barbs.

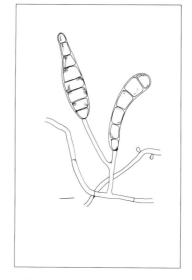

Figure 52.1 *Microsporum gallinae.*

150

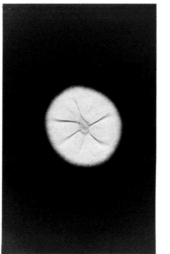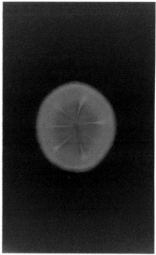

Figure 52.2   Sabouraud glucose agar, 25°C,
7 days (surface/reverse).

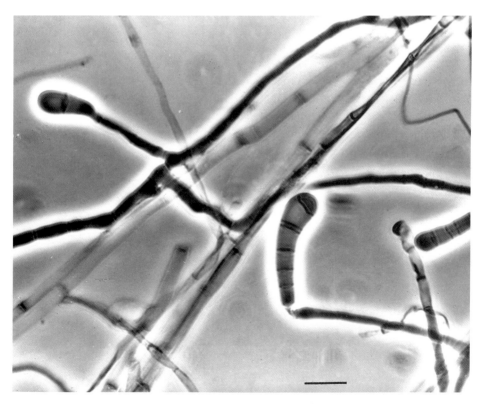

Figure 52.3   *Microsporum gallinae*. Curved macroconidia.
(Courtesy of L. Sigler).

Microsporum gypseum   (Bodin) Guiart et Grigorakis, 1928

Pathogenicity: occasionally a cause of infection of the scalp or the glabrous skin in humans. Infected hairs show little or no fluorescence under the Wood's light. A great variety of animals are infected or carry the organism.

Ecology: a cosmopolitan geophilic dermatophyte, frequently isolated from soil and from the fur of small rodents.

Colony appearance:
- rapid growth;
- texture downy becoming powdery to granular;
- color beige on the surface; reverse beige to red brown.

Microscopic appearance:
- macroconidia typically abundant, ellipsoidal to fusiform, symmetrical, thin-walled, containing 3 to 6 cells;
- microconidia moderately abundant, club-shaped.

Physiological tests:
- hair perforation: positive
- growth factor requirements: none
- BCP-milk solids-glucose: no change in pH

Remarks: *M. gypseum* produces powdery beige colonies with numerous symmetrical, thin-walled macroconidia. *Microsporum fulvum* and *M. gypseum* are closely related members of the *M. gypseum* complex. For definitive identification of members of this complex, mating trials *in vitro* with reference mating test strains are necessary. *Microsporum praecox*, on the other hand, can be distinguished by its colonies with yellow reverse, and longer macroconidia composed of 6 to 9 cells; moreover, it does not perforate hair *in vitro*.

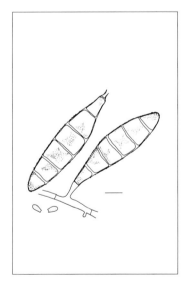

Figure 53.1   *Microsporum gypseum.*

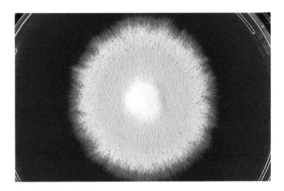

Figure 53.2   Sabouraud glucose agar,
25°C, 7 days.

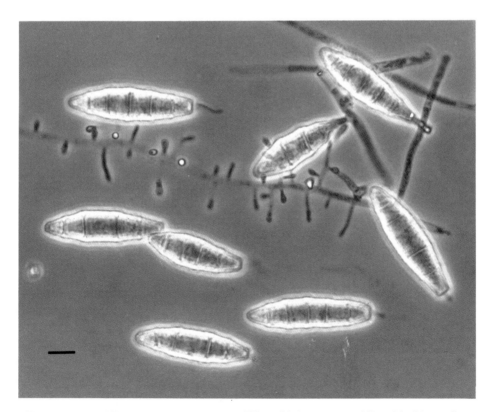

Figure 53.3   *Microsporum gypseum*. Ellipsoidal macroconidia with thin walls.

Microsporum nanum Fuentes, 1956

Pathogenicity: principal cause of tinea of the pig. The infection is rarely transmitted to humans.

Ecology: cosmopolitan dermatophyte, geophilic and zoophilic, commonly associated with swine.

Colony appearance:
- moderately rapid growth;
- texture powdery;
- color white to yellowish on the surface; reverse red brown.

Microscopic appearance:
- microconidia club-shaped, numerous to rare;
- macroconidia ovoid to ellipsoidal, normally with only 2 cells.

Physiological tests:
- hair perforation: positive
- growth factor requirements: none

Remarks: *Microsporum nanum* is distinguished by its typically ovoid macroconidia normally containing only 2 cells. Unlike the *Trichothecium*, its conidia are solitary on the ends of short conidiophores and its growth is not inhibited by cycloheximide in Mycosel agar.

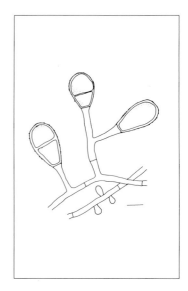

Figure 54.1 *Micro-sporum nanum.*

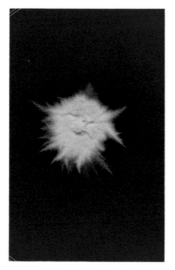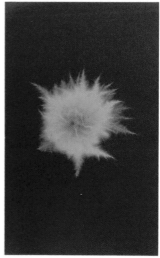

Figure 54.2   Sabouraud glucose agar, 25°C,
7 days (surface/reverse).

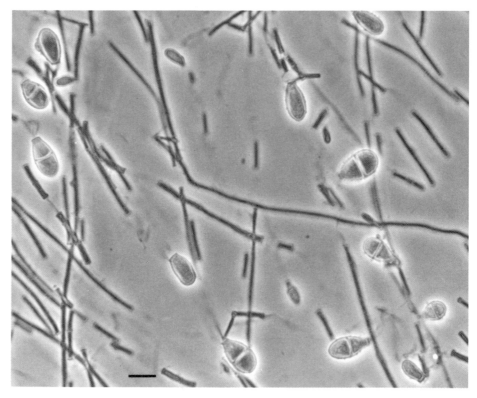

Figure 54.3   *Microsporum nanum.* Macroconidia with 2 cells.

Microsporum persicolor
(Sabouraud) Guiart et Grigorakis, 1928

Pathogenicity: a sporadic cause of infection of the scalp, the glabrous skin and the feet in humans. Animal infection, principally associated with certain rodents and bats, is also sometimes found in dogs.

Ecology: cosmopolitan, a zoophilic dermatophyte having its principal reservoir in small rodents such as the vole and the field mouse.

Colony appearance:
- rapid growth;
- texture downy to powdery;
- color yellowish to rosy on the surface; reverse uncolored, pink or red brown.

Microscopic appearance:
- spiral hyphae frequent;
- microconidia numerous, club-shaped or round, often pedicellate;
- macroconidia often present in primary isolates, fusiform or bullet shaped, with smooth walls, lightly roughened at the tips, often containing 6 cells.

Physiological tests:
- hair perforation: positive
- growth factor requirements: none
- growth at 37°C: weak
- BCP-milk solids-glucose: no change of pH

Remarks: unlike *Trichophyton mentagrophytes*, M. persicolor grows poorly at 37°C and fails to produce an alkaline reaction on BCP-milk solids-glucose. The colony reverse takes on a characteristic pinkish hue when the organism is grown on peptone agar without sugar. Its microconidia are often produced at the end of pedicels. Freshly isolated strains produce fusiform or bullet-shaped macroconidia. The formation of numerous rough- walled macroconidia can be stimulated by growing colonies on Sabouraud glucose agar containing 3% to 5% sodium chloride.

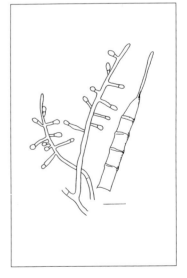

Figure 55.1   *Microsporum persicolor.*

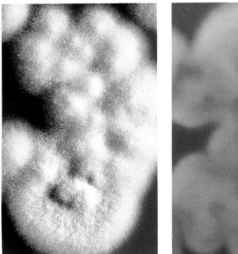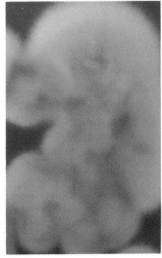

Figure 55.2   Sabouraud glucose agar, 25°C,
21 days (surface/reverse).

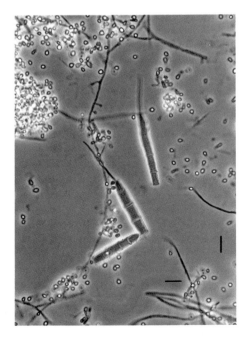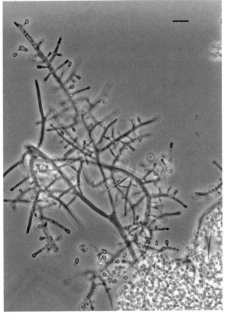

Figure 55.3   *Microsporum persicolor*. A, Fusiform macroconidia, some with a
flagelliform appendage at the tip. B, Pedicellate microconidia.

Mucor

Micheli ex Fries, 1832

Pathogenicity: uncommonly an agent of zygomycosis in the severely debilitated patient.

Ecology: cosmopolitan, saprobic, coprophilic, isolated from decaying organic material and from most normal stool specimens.

Colony appearance:
- very rapid growth;
- texture wooly;
- color greyish to brownish on the surface; reverse pale.

Microscopic appearance:
- hyphae broad, not or scarcely septate;
- sporangiophores branched or sometimes unbranched;
- sporangia with columellas, lacking apophyses;
- sporangiospores round to ellipsoidal;
- chlamydospores sometimes present;
- rhizoids and stolons absent.

Remarks: *Mucor* differs from *Rhizopus* in not producing rhizoids, and from *Absidia* by the absence of an apophysis beneath the sporangium. In contrast to *Rhizomucor*, the maximum temperature for growth in *Mucor* is well below 54°C; the great majority of species are unable to grow at 37°C.

Bibliography:
Domsch, Gams, Anderson, 1980
Kwon-Chung, Bennett, 1992
Scholer, Müller, Schipper, 1983

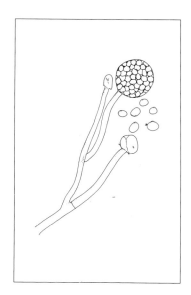

Figure 56.1   *Mucor* sp.

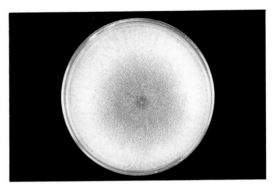

Figure 56.2   Potato glucose agar,
25°C, 7 days.

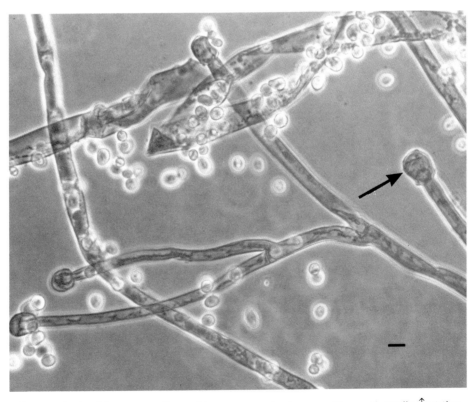

Figure 56.3   *Mucor* sp. Branching sporangiophores with a columella $^\uparrow$ at the
tip; the sporangia, having dispersed their spores into the
aqueous mounting medium, are no longer in evidence.

159

Nigrospora

Zimmerman, 1902

Pathogenicity: no cases of infection have been recorded in humans or animals.

Ecology: cosmopolitan, saprobes isolated from decaying plant material and soil.

Colony appearance:
- growth rapid to very rapid;
- texture wooly;
- color white becoming black on surface and reverse.

Microscopic appearance:
- hyphae septate, hyaline;
- conidiophores hyaline, short and inflated;
- conidia black, unicellular, ovoid to ellipsoidal, slightly horizontally flattened (oblate), smooth walled, with a thin equatorial germ slit.

Remarks: *Nigrospora* produces black conidia, slightly but distinctly horizontally flattened, supported by short, centrally inflated conidiophores. Certain isolates require more than 3 weeks of incubation before they sporulate.

Bibliography:
Domsch, Gams, Anderson, 1980

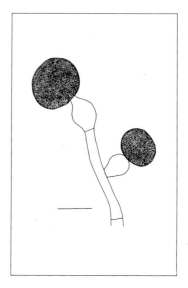

Figure 57.1 *Nigrospora* sp.

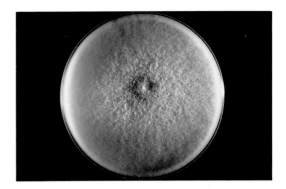

Figure 57.2   Potato glucose agar,
25°C, 7 days.

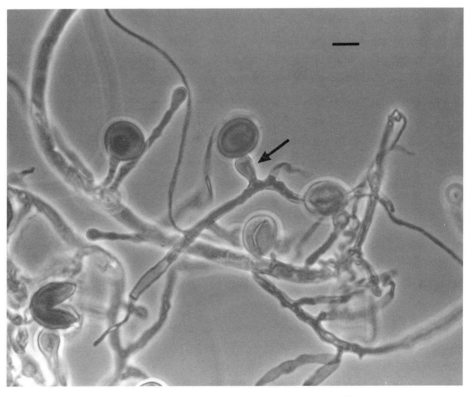

Figure 57.3   *Nigrospora* sp. Black, ovoid conidia, produced on an inflated
conidiophore↑.

Paecilomyces

Bainier, 1907

Pathogenicity: relatively rarely pathogenic in humans. Among the cases reported are instances of keratitis associated with corneal implants, endocarditis diagnosed after valve replacement surgery, peritonitis in dialysis patients, as well as a few cases of cellulitis or pneumonia in the immunocompromised patient.

Ecology: cosmopolitan, isolated from soil and decaying plant material. Often implicated in decay of food products and cosmetics. Certain species parasitize insects.

Colony appearance:
- rapid growth;
- texture wooly to powdery;
- color rusty, olive brown, lilac, pinkish, beige or white on the surface; reverse pale.

Microscopic appearance:
- hyphae septate, hyaline;
- conidiophores often branched;
- phialides thin and elongate at the tips, grouped in brush-like clusters at the ends of the conidiophores;
- conidia oval to fusoid, in long chains;
- chlamydospores sometimes present.

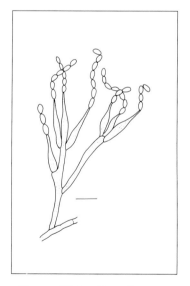

Remarks: *Paecilomyces* is distinguished from *Penicillium* by its phialides with thin, elongate tips, often slightly splayed apart. *Penicillium*, by contrast, has phialides with thicker apices and these apices tend to have a nearly parallel orientation in tight clusters. Also, unlike most species of *Penicillium*, *Paecilomyces* never has blue or green colonies.

Bibliography:
Domsch, Gams, Anderson, 1980
Kwon-Chung, Bennett, 1992
McGinnis, 1980
Samson, 1974

Figure 58.1 *Paecilo-myces* sp.

162

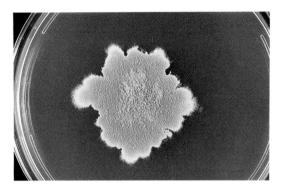

Figure 58.2 *Paecilomyces variotii.*
Potato glucose agar,
25°C, 7 days.

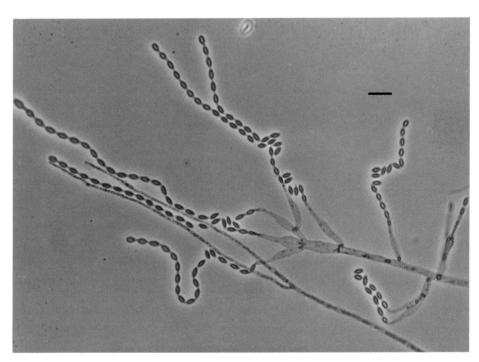

Figure 58.3 *Paecilomyces variotii.* Phialides with thinly tapered apices and chains of oval conidia.

Paracoccidioides brasiliensis de Almeida, 1930

Pathogenicity: *Paracoc-cidioides brasiliensis* is the etio-logic agent of paracoccidioi-domycosis. This chronic illness, acquired via inhalation, may remain asymptomatic or progress in the form of a pul-monary or disseminated infec-tion, usually producing secon-dary lesions of the buccal, nasal or gastrointestinal mucosa.

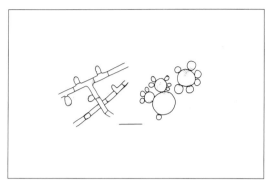

Figure 59.1 *Paracoccidioides brasiliensis.* Filamentous form at 25°C and yeast form at 37°C.

Ecology: *P. brasiliensis* has been isolated only on a few occasions from non-medical sources, chiefly soil and the digestive tracts of animals, and its exact habitat remains unknown. Its geographic distribution is restricted to South America where the majority of cases are diagnosed in Brazil, Venezuela, and Colombia.

DIMORPHIC FUNGUS

Colony appearance:

at 25°C:

- slow to very slow growth
- texture glabrous to velvety;
- color white, pink, beige or brown on the surface with reverse yellowish to brown.

at 37°C, on rich medium:

- very slow growth
- texture creamy
- color white

Microscopic appearance:

at 25°C:

- hyphae septate, hyaline, often sterile;
- aleurioconidia, arthroconidia and chlamydospores often present, but not a distinctive feature of the species.

at 37°C, on rich medium or in infected tissues:

- yeasts with multiple "satellite" budding.

Remarks: freshly isolated strains may sometimes sporulate weakly on cul-ture media commonly used in medical mycology, but the majority of cultures are sterile. For this reason certain biological safety manuals have now removed

164

this species from their lists of the most highly biohazardous fungi in the laboratory environment. *P. brasiliensis* is recognized by its yeasts with multiple buds, induced at 37°C on rich media.

Bibliography:

Kwon-Chung, Bennett, 1992
McGinnis, 1980
Rippon, 1988

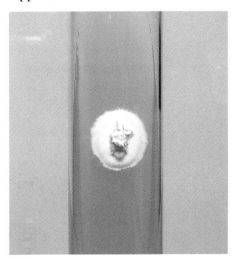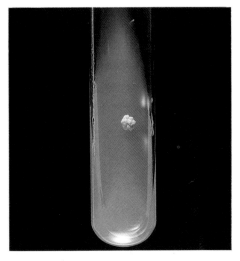

Figure 59.2   A, Filamentous form on Sabouraud glucose agar, 25°C, 21 days. B, Yeast form on brain-heart infusion agar, 37°C, 21 days.

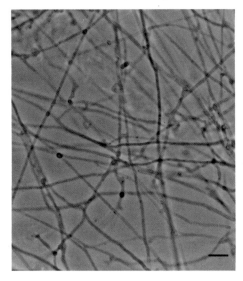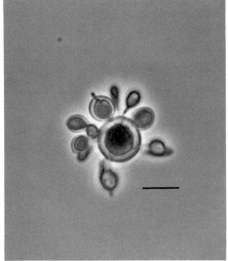

Figure 59.3   *Paracoccidioides brasiliensis.* A, Hyphae with some arthroconidia at 25°C. B, Yeast with multiple buds at 37°C.

Penicillium

Pathogenicity: normally nonpathogenic with the exception of *Penicillium marneffei*, a dimorphic species capable of causing infection of the lymphatic system, the lungs, the liver, the skin, the spleen, and the bones.

Ecology: cosmopolitan, predominant in regions of temperate climate. Penicillia figure among the most common types of fungi isolated from the environment. Of the approximately 150 species recognized, some are frequently implicated in the deterioration of food products, where they may elaborate mycotoxins. Other species are producers of penicillin. Infections with *P. marneffei* are primarily acquired in mountainous provinces of northern Thailand, Laos, Myanmar, and southeastern China.

Colony appearance:
- growth moderately rapid to rapid;
- texture velvety to powdery;
- color green, blue-green, grey-green, white, yellow, or pinkish on the surface; reverse usually pale to yellowish, sometimes red or brown.

Microscopic appearance:
- hyphae septate, hyaline;
- conidiophores simple or branched;
- phialides grouped in brush-like clusters (penicilli) at the ends of the conidiophores;
- conidia unicellular, round to ovoid, hyaline or pigmented, rough walled or smooth, in chains.

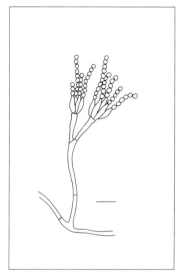

Figure 60.1   *Penicillium* sp.

Remarks: *Penicillium* is distinguished by its frequently greenish colonies and its branching or simple conidiophores supporting phialides in brush-like clusters known as penicilli. It is differentiated from *Paecilomyces* by its phialides lacking long, pointed apical extensions. In contrast to *Scopulariopsis*, its conidia lack a truncate base. *P. marneffei* produces downy grey-green colonies, often with a brownish or red tint caused by the presence of red or yellow pigmented sterile hyphae in the colony. A red pigment characteristically diffuses into the medium. At 37°C on Sabouraud glucose agar, the colonies characteristically lose this pigmentation and convert into yeast-like cells multiplying by fission. The diagnosis of infection due to *P. marneffei* rests on the histopathologic demonstration of cells multiplying by fission in the interior of leukocytes.

166

Bibliography:
Domsch, Gams,
   Anderson, 1980
Drouhet, 1993
Kwon-Chung, Bennett, 1992

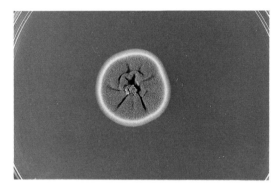

Figure 60.2   *Penicillium* sp.
Potato glucose agar,
25°C, 7 days.

Figure 60.3   *Penicillium* sp.
Phialides
grouped in
brush-like
penicilli and
producing
conidia in chains.

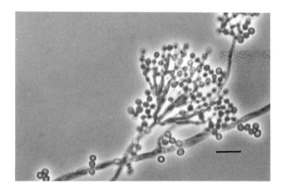

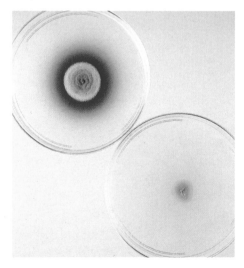

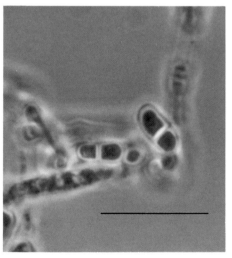

Figure 60.4   *Penicillium marneffei*. A, Sabouraud glucose agar, 25°C and
37°C, 7 days. B, Cells multiplying by fission in culture at 37°C
on Sabouraud glucose agar.

Phialophora Medlar, 1915

Pathogenicity: the genus *Phialophora* includes *P. verrucosa*, one of the agents of chromoblastomycosis. It also includes several species causing diverse types of phaeohyphomycosis, presenting in the form of mycotic arthritis, subcutaneous cyst, osteomyelitis, and cerebral or disseminated infection.

Ecology: cosmopolitan, saprobes commonly isolated from decomposing wood, soil, and subaquatic debris in bodies of cold fresh water.

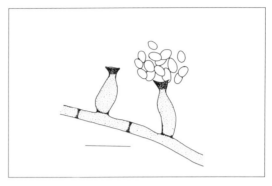

Figure 61.1 *Phialophora verrucosa.*

Colony appearance:
- slow growth;
- texture velvety to wooly;
- color dark grey, brown or black on surface and reverse.

Microscopic appearance:
- hyphae septate, hyaline to brown;
- phialides pale brown to brown, bottle-shaped or cylindrical, with a collarette at the tip;
- conidia unicellular, hyaline or brown, round, ovoid, cylindrical or curved, typically accumulating at the tips of phialides in slimy masses.

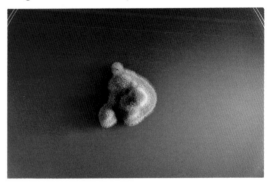

Figure 61.2 *Phialophora verrucosa.*
Potato glucose agar, 25°C, 7 days.

Remarks: *Phialophora* is distinguished from *Exophiala* a n d *Wangiella dermatitidis* by its phialides with readily visible collarettes. The shape of the collarettes is important in identification of the medically important species: those of *Phialophora verrucosa* are vase-shaped, those of *P. richardsiae* are saucer-shaped and vase-shaped,

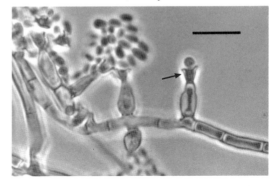

Figure 61.3 Phialides with vase-shaped collarette[↑].

168

and those of P. repens and P. parasitica are narrow, with nearly parallel sides in optical section. The phialides of *P. parasitica* are long (often > 20 μm) and narrowly spine-shaped, while those of *P. repens* are shorter (often < 20 μm) and sometimes sinuous and lacking a septum at the base. *P. parasitica* also typically produces hyphae with verrucose walls.

Bibliography:

Dixon, Polak-Wyss, 1991
Domsch, Gams,
  Anderson, 1980
de Hoog, 1983
Kwon-Chung, Bennett, 1992
McGinnis, 1980

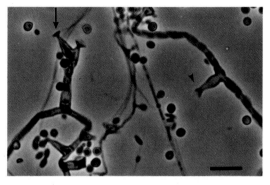

Figure 61.4   *Phialophora richardsiae.* Phialides with saucer-shaped collarette↑ producing round conidia, and phialides with vase-shaped collarettes▲ producing cylindrical conidia.

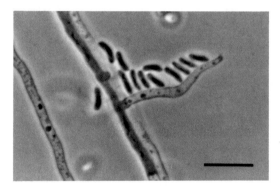

Figure 61.5   *Phialophora repens.* Cylindrical, sinuous phialide.

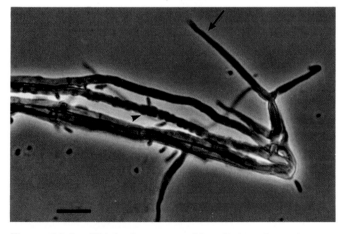

Figure 61.6   *Phialophora parasitica.* Spine-shaped phialides↑ and hyphae with rough walls▲.

Phoma Saccardo, 1880, nom. cons.

Pathogenicity: in exceptional cases a cause of infection in humans or animals. To date, only a few cases of subcutaneous phaeohyphomycosis have been reported.

Ecology: cosmopolitan, common plant pathogens, frequently isolated from soil.

Colony appearance:
- rapid growth;
- texture powdery to velvety;
- surface color olive grey, sometimes with a tint of pink; reverse dark brown, with a brown diffusible pigment in some species.

Microscopic appearance:
- hyphae septate, hyaline or brown;
- pycnidia round to pyriform, ostiolate, brown to black;
- conidia hyaline, unicellular, ellipsoidal to cylindrical.

Remarks: *Phoma* produces olive grey colonies and pycnidia which, at maturity, liberate conidia through an opening called an ostiole. It must not be confused with other similarly colored fungi which produce ascospores within perithecia or cleistothecia, such as *Chaetomium* or *Pseudallescheria boydii*.

Bibliography:
Domsch, Gams, Anderson, 1980
Kwon-Chung, Bennett, 1992
McGinnis, 1980
Rippon, 1988

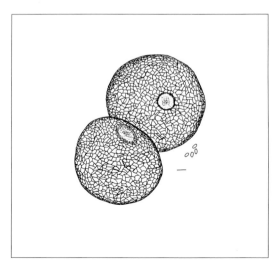

Figure 62.1 *Phoma* sp.

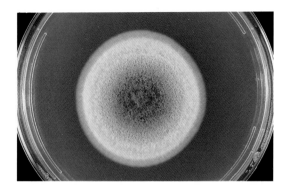

Figure 62.2   Potato glucose agar,
25°C, 7 days.

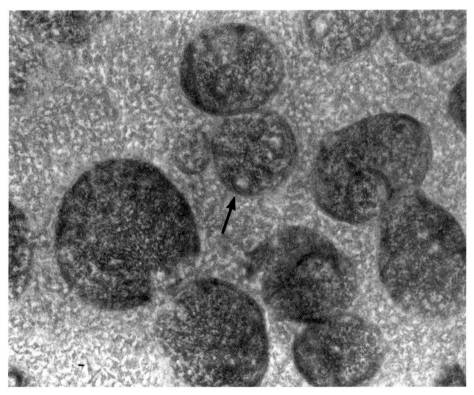

Figure 62.3   *Phoma* sp. Ostiolate[↑] pycnidia.

Pithomyces

Berkeley et Broome, 1873

Pathogenicity: no cases of infection have been reported in humans or animals.

Ecology: cosmopolitan, saprobes isolated from decaying wood or other plant material and from soil.

Colony appearance:
- very rapid growth;
- texture wooly to flocculent;
- color pale to dark grey or brown on the surface; reverse dark brown.

Microscopic appearance:
- hyphae septate, hyaline or brown;
- conidiophores hardly differentiated from vegetative hyphae;
- conidia muriform, brown, ellipsoidal to club-shaped, with smooth or roughened wall, borne singly.

Remarks: *Pithomyces* differs from *Alternaria* and *Ulocladium* by its scarcely differentiated conidiophores, and its conidia (aleurioconidia) which, once liberated, retain an annular frill at the base. It never produces conidia in chains. A good proportion of isolates fail to sporulate on conventional media; their sporulation can be induced by culture on 2% agar or soil extract agar.

Bibliography:
Domsch, Gams, Anderson, 1980

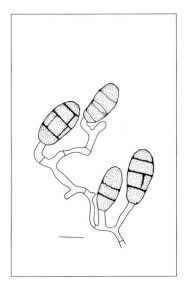

Figure 63.1   *Pithomyces* sp.

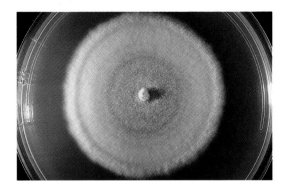

Figure 63.2   Potato glucose agar,
25°C, 7 days.

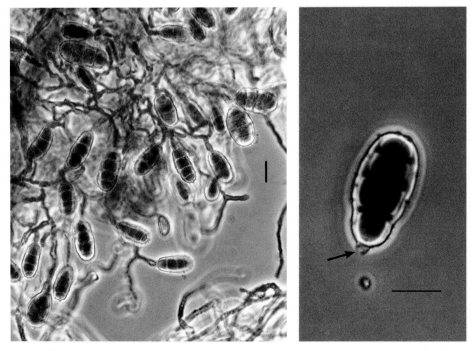

Figure 63.3   *Pithomyces* sp. A, Muriform conidia, produced singly on
minimally differentiated conidiophores. B, Annular frill[↑].

173

Rhinocladiella Nannfeldt, 1934

Pathogenicity: to date, only 3 cases of subcutaneous infection caused by *Rhinocladiella aquaspersa* have been reported from humans.

Ecology: cosmopolitan, isolated from decaying wood.

Colony appearance:
- growth slow to moderately rapid;
- texture velvety;
- color olive black on surface and reverse.

Microscopic appearance:
- hyphae septate, brown;
- conidiophores cylindrical, brown, unbranched;
- conidia ellipsoidal to club-shaped, mostly unicellular or sometimes bicellular, pale brown, borne on denticles, arranged in a closely spaced series at and beneath the apex of the conidiophore.

Remarks: *Rhinocladiella* is distinguished by its olive black colonies and its ellipsoidal conidia disposed in a thinly plume- like arrangement at the end of an unbranched conidiophore. Unlike *Fonsecaea*, *Rhinocladiella* does not have secondary ranks of conidia arising out of the conidia that form initially. Only a single rank of conidia is seen at the apex of the conidiophore. Note, however, that *Rhinocladiella* states are also occasionally seen in polymorphous fungi such as *Exophiala* and *Fonsecaea*.

Bibliography:
de Hoog, 1983
Kwon-Chung, Bennett, 1992
Schell, McGinnis, 1988

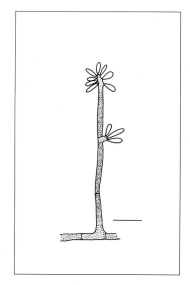

Figure 64.1   *Rhino-cladiella* sp.

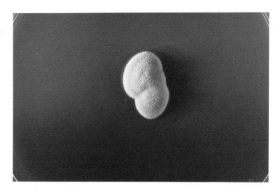

Figure 64.2   Potato glucose agar, 25°C, 7 days.

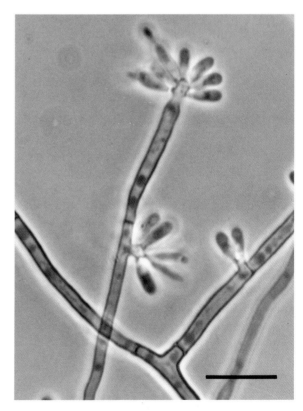

Figure 64.3   *Rhinocladiella* sp. Ellipsoidal conidia arranged in a plume-like series at the apex of a conidiophore.

175

Rhizomucor (Lucet et Constantin) Wehmer ex Vuillemin, 1931

Pathogenicity: *Rhizomucor pusillus* is occasionally an agent of pulmonary, rhinofacial, cerebral or disseminated zygomycosis. So far, infections have mainly been encountered in the leukemic patient.

Ecology: cosmopolitan, thermophilic, often isolated from composting or fermenting organic matter.

Colony appearance:
- rapid growth;
- texture wooly;
- color pale brown on the surface; reverse white.

Microscopic appearance:
- hyphae broad, not or scarcely septate;
- rudimentary rhizoids and stolons present but often rare or difficult to recognize;
- sporangiophores branched, with branches sometimes arranged in an umbel at the apex;
- apophysis absent;
- sporangia round with well developed columella;
- sporangiospores round or oval.

Remarks: *Rhizomucor* differs from *Mucor* by its tolerance of high growth temperatures (≥ 54°C) and by the presence of occasional rhizoids and stolons. In contrast to *Absidia*, *Rhizomucor* does not possess an apophysis, and unlike *Rhizopus*, it generally has branched sporangiophores and comparatively rare, poorly developed rhizoids. *Rhizomucor (Mucor) pusillus* is the only species known as a pathogen.

Bibliography:
Domsch, Gams, Anderson, 1980
Kwon-Chung, Bennett, 1992
Scholer, Müller, Schipper, 1983

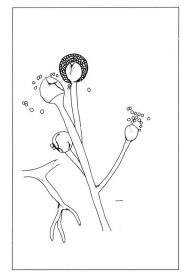

Figure 65.1 *Rhizomucor pusillus.*

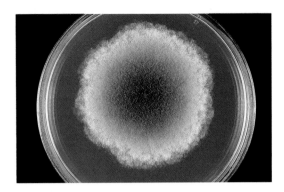

Figure 65.2   *Rhizomucor pusillus*.
Potato glucose agar,
25°C, 7 days.

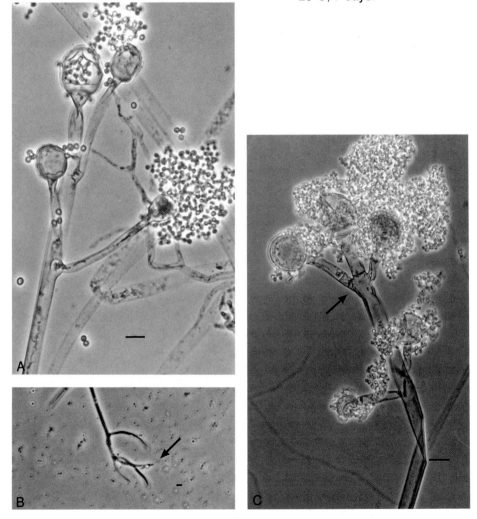

Figure 65.3   *Rhizomucor pusillus*. A, Branched sporangiophore.
B, Rudimentary rhizoids. C, Umbellate sporangiophore.

Rhizopus Ehrenberg, 1820

Pathogenicity: *Rhizopus* is the principal agent of zygomycosis. This rapidly progressing infection is characterized by the necrosis of tissues and the production of infarcts in the brain, the lungs, and the intestines. Primarily, it is patients suffering from diabetic ketoacidosis, malnutrition, severe burns, or immunocompromising conditions who are most at risk to develop this type of infection.

Ecology: cosmopolitan, frequently isolated from soil and agricultural products (cereals, vegetables, etc.). Certain species are plant pathogens.

Colony appearance:
- very rapid growth;
- texture deeply cottony;
- color white becoming grey brown on the surface; reverse pale.

Microscopic appearance:
- hyphae broad, not or scarcely septate;
- rhizoids and stolons present;
- sporangiophores brown, solitary or in tufts on the stolons, diverging from the point at which the rhizoids form;
- sporangia rather round;
- apophysis absent or scarcely apparent;
- sporangiospores ovoid.

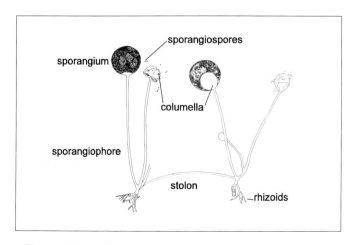

Figure 66.1   *Rhizopus* sp.

Remarks: *Rhizopus* is recognized by the presence of well developed rhizoids situated at the point where sporangiophores are attached to the stolons. In contrast to *Mucor*, *Rhizomucor* and *Absidia*, the sporangiophores are often unbranched and grouped in tufts.

Bibliography:

Domsch, Gams,
 Anderson, 1980
Kwon-Chung, Bennett, 1992
Scholer, Müller, Schipper, 1983

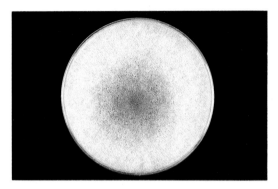

Figure 66.2   Potato glucose agar, 25°C, 7 days.

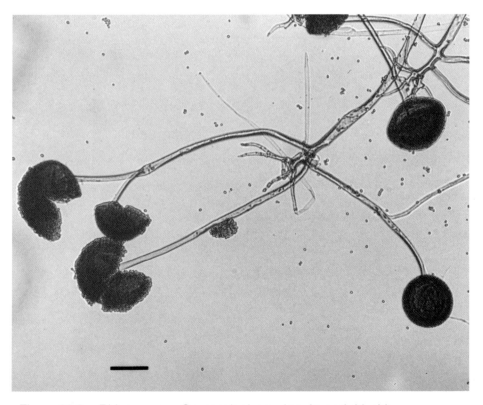

Figure 66.3   *Rhizopus* sp. Sporangiophores in tufts and rhizoids.

Scedosporium apiospermum

Saccardo ex Castellani et Chalmers, 1919

= *Monosporium apiospermum*
Teleomorph = *Pseudallescheria boydii*

Pathogenicity: an occasional agent of infections including mycetoma, cutaneous or subcutaneous invasion, otitis, sinusitis, keratitis, endophthalmitis, pneumonia, endocarditis, meningitis, osteomyelitis, cerebral abscess and disseminated infection. Systemic infection is more commonly seen in the debilitated patient than in the normal host, but may occur in the latter under certain circumstances.

Ecology: cosmopolitan, commonly isolated from rural soils, from polluted water, from composts, and from manure of cattle and fowl.

Colony appearance:
- rapid growth;
- texture wooly to cottony;
- color white becoming brownish on the surface; reverse pale with brownish black zones.

Figure 67.1 Cleisthotecium of the sexual state *Pseudallescheria boydii* ; conidia of the asexual state *Scedosporium apiospermum*.

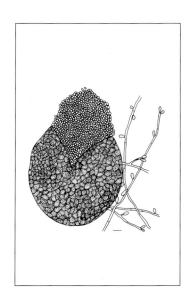

180

Microscopic appearance:
- hyphae septate, hyaline;
- conidiophores with annellides simple or branched, little differentiated from vegetative hyphae;
- conidia (annelloconidia) unicellular, pale brown, obovoid, with truncate bases, formed singly or in small clusters at the ends of conidiophores or from short annellidic necks arising directly from the hyphae (*Scedosporium* asexual state, always present);
- fascicles of conidiophores bound together in synnemata sometimes present (*Graphium* state);
- brown cleistothecia often present after 2-3 weeks of incubation (sexual state *Pseudallescheria boydii*);
- ascospores yellow-brown, ellipsoidal.

Remarks: *S. apiospermum* is the asexual state of a homothallic fungus, *P. boydii*. Since some isolates appear to lack the ability to complete the homothallic sexual process and form cleistothecia, the name of the consistently seen asexual state is used here in preference. *S. apiospermum* produces unicellular, brown annelloconidia with truncate bases. *Scedosporium prolificans* (= *S. inflatum*) is distinguished from *S. apiospermum* by its basally inflated annellides, its growth at 45°C and its inhibition by cycloheximide in Mycosel agar. It has no known sexual state. Unlike *Sporothrix schenckii* and *Blastomyces dermatitidis*, *Scedosporium* species do not convert to a yeast phase at 37°C on rich media.

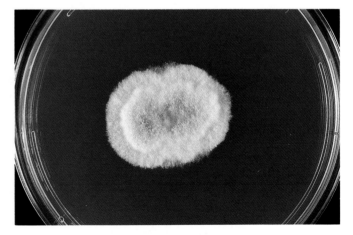

Figure 67.2 *Scedosporium apiospermum.*
Potato glucose agar, 25°C, 7 days.

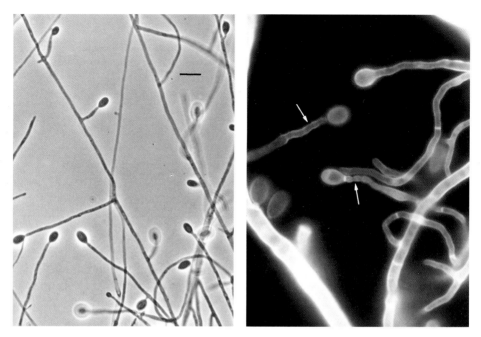

Figure 67.3   *Scedosporium apiospermum.* A, Conidia at the tips of more or less elongate conidiophores. B, Annellides with annular rings (fluorescence/calcofluor white).

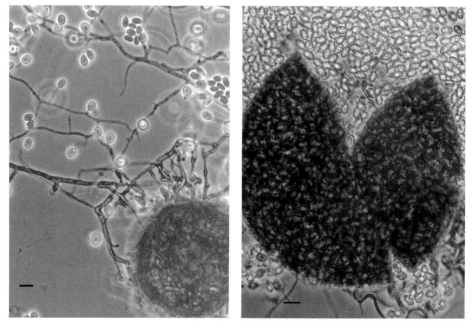

Figure 67.4   *Pseudallescheria boydii.* A, Cleistothecia releasing ellipsoidal ascospores. B, Immature cleistothecia and conidia of the *Scedosporium* state.

Bibliography:
Gueho, de Hoog, 1991
Kwon-Chung, Bennett, 1992
McGinnis, Padhye, Ajello 1982

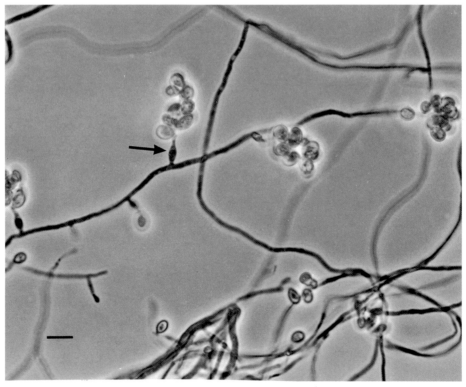

Figure 67.5   *Scedosporium prolificans*.   Basally inflated annellides[↑].

Scolecobasidium

Abbott, 1927

= *Ochroconis* (de Hoog, von Arx, 1974)

Pathogenicity: no cases of infection have been reported from humans. A few cases of phaeohyphomycosis have been reported in fish, namely coho salmon and rainbow trout.

Ecology: cosmopolitan, principally soil saprobes.

Colony appearance:
- slow growth;
- texture velvety to flocculent;
- color brown on surface and reverse.

Microscopic appearance:
- hyphae septate, pale brown;
- conidiophores brown, unbranched, with apical denticles in a sympodial arrangement;
- conidia pale brown, cylindrical to club shaped, with one or several transverse septa.

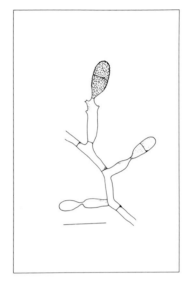

Figure 68.1   *Scoleco-basidium* sp.

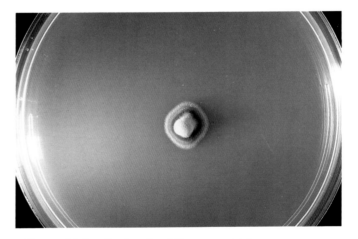

Figure 68.2   *Scolecobasidium constrictum.*
Potato glucose agar, 25°C, 7 days.

Remarks: the taxonomic status of *Scolecobasidium, Ochroconis* and *Dactylaria* remains the subject of controversy. *Scolecobasidium constrictum* and *Dactylaria gallopava* produce morphologically similar, bicellular conidia. *S. constrictum* does not grow at 37°C and is resistant to cycloheximide, while *D. gallopava* produces violaceous brown colonies, grows more rapidly at 37°C than at 30°C, and is inhibited on Mycosel agar. *D. gallopava* is rarely a cause of subcutaneous or disseminated infection in the immunocompromised patient; it is also responsible for outbreaks of acute encephalitis in fowl.

Bibliography:

Domsch, Gams,
   Anderson, 1980
de Hoog, 1983
Kwon-Chung,
   Bennett, 1992

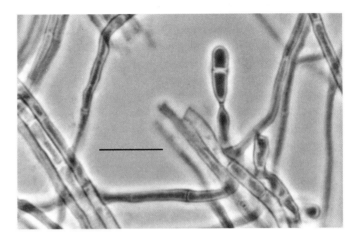

Figure 68.3   *Scolecobasidium constrictum.*
Unbranched conidiophore with
bicellular conidia formed on a denticle.

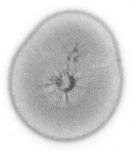

Figure 68.4   *Dactylaria gallopava.*
Brown violet colony
growing strongly at 37°C
(Sabouraud glucose agar,
7 days).

Scopulariopsis
Bainier, 1907

Pathogenicity: rarely a cause of human infection. Onychomycosis is occasionally reported, while reports of subcutaneous and pulmonary infection are rare, and primarily concern the immunocompromised host.

Ecology: cosmopolitan, frequently isolated from soil. Certain species attack bee larvae and silkworms.

Colony appearance:
- moderately rapid growth;
- texture velvety to powdery;
- color white, cinnamon, greyish or black on the surface; reverse yellowish to black.

Microscopic appearance:
- hyphae septate, hyaline or dark;
- conidiophores with annellides hyaline or dark, simple or branched;
- conidia hyaline or dark grey, unicellular, pyriform with truncate bases, smooth or rough walled, in chains.

Remarks: *Scopulariopsis* species are frequently isolated in the clinical laboratory. Unlike *Penicillium*, they produce pyriform conidia, typically with truncate bases. *Scopulariopsis brevicaulis* is recognized by its cinnamon colored colonies and its long cylindrical conidiophores, often clustered together in penicillus-like structures. *Scopulariopsis brumptii* is distinguished by its grey to grey black colonies and its short, swollen conidiophores.

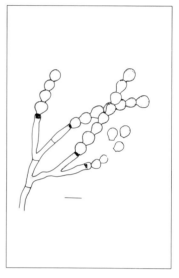

Figure 69.1   *Scopulariopsis brevicaulis.*

Bibliography:
Domsch, Gams,
  Anderson, 1980
Kwon-Chung, Bennett, 1992

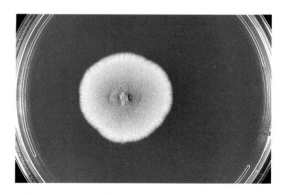

Figure 69.2   *Scopulariopsis brevicaulis.*
Potato glucose agar,
25°C, 7 days.

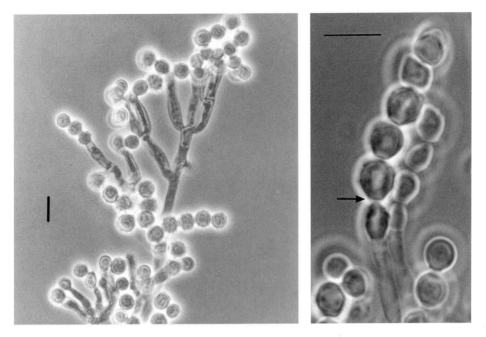

Figure 69.3 *Scopulariopsis brevicaulis*. A, Branched conidiophores and conidia in chains. B, Pyriform conidia with truncate bases[↑].

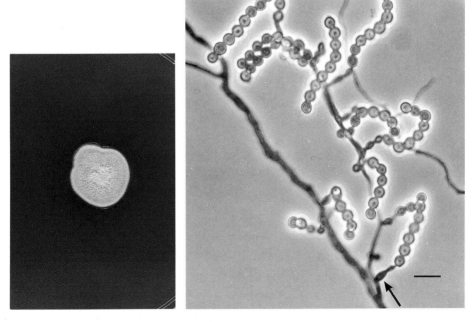

Figure 69.4 *Scopulariopsis brumptii*. A, Potato glucose agar, 25°C, 7 days. B, Conidiophore with inflated base.

Scytalidium Pesante, 1957

Pathogenicity: occasionally an agent of nail or skin infection. Some cases of subcutaneous or disseminated infection have also been noted.

Ecology: cosmopolitan saprobes, sometimes associated with decaying wood or with soil, sometimes with diseases of woody plants, especially in tropical and subtropical regions.

Colony appearance:
- very rapid growth;
- texture wooly;
- color white to grey black on the surface and on the reverse.

Microscopic appearance:
- hyphae septate, hyaline or pale grey;
- conidiophores absent;
- arthroconidia hyaline or pale brown, unicellular or bicellular, oval or ellipsoidal.

Remarks: *Scytalidium* is distinguished from *Geotrichum* by its wooly colonies and, in most species, by its brown pigmented hyphae and arthroconidia. *Scytalidium dimidiatum* produces brown arthroconidia and also possesses a pycnidial state known by the name *Nattrassia mangiferae* (= *Hendersonula toruloidea*). *Scytalidium hyalinum* produces hyaline arthroconidia. These two species are agents of onychomycosis and dermatomycosis. They are usually inhibited by cycloheximide and cannot be isolated on Mycosel agar.

Bibliography:
Kwon-Chung, Bennett, 1992
McGinnis, 1980
Moore, 1988
Sutton, Dyko, 1989

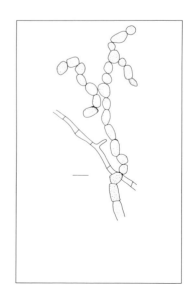

Figure 70.1
Scytalidium
sp.

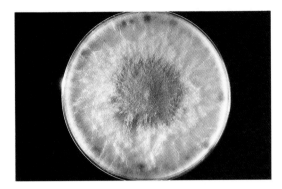

Figure 70.2 *Scytalidium dimidiatum*.
Potato glucose agar,
25°C, 7 days.

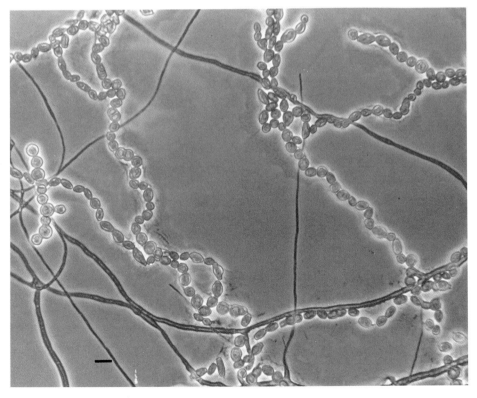

Figure 70.3 *Scytalidium dimidiatum*.   Brown arthroconidia.

189

Sepedonium

Pathogenicity: no cases of infection have been reported in humans or animals.

Ecology: cosmopolitan, soil saprobes and parasites of mushrooms in the order Boletales.

Colony appearance:
- rapid growth;
- texture wooly;
- color white to golden yellow on the surface; reverse pale.

Microscopic appearance:
- hyphae septate, hyaline;
- conidiophores little differentiated from vegetative hyphae;
- conidia unicellular, terminal, solitary, rather rounded, thick- walled, often echinulate or verrucose;
- a phialidic conidial state producing ellipsoidal or cylindrical, smooth walled conidia also sometimes present at the beginning of colony growth.

Remarks: *Sepedonium* may resemble *Histoplasma capsulatum* but is usually distinguished by the absence of microaleurioconidia and by its more rapid colonial growth. In cases of doubt, the inability of *Sepedonium* to convert to a yeast phase at 37°C on rich media and its negative test in exoantigen or probe trials specific for *H. capsulatum* can be used to avoid confusion with the dimorphic fungal pathogen.

Bibliography:
Domsch, Gams, Anderson, 1980 (see entry for *Hypomyces*)
Kwon-Chung, Bennett, 1992
McGinnis, 1980

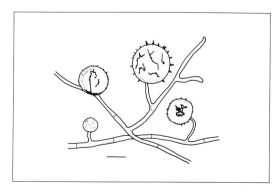

Figure 71.1 *Sepedonium* sp.

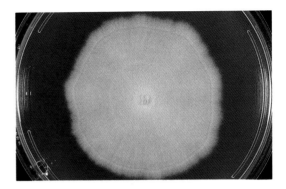

Figure 71.2   Potato glucose agar,
25°C, 7 days.

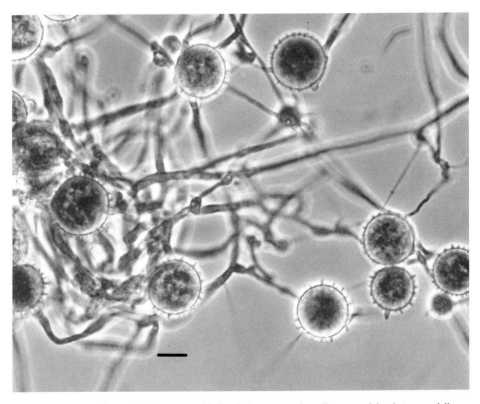

Figure 71.3   *Sepedonium* sp. Unicellular, round, solitary, echinulate conidia.

Sporothrix schenckii

Hektoen et Perkins, 1900

Pathogenicity: *Sporothrix schenckii* is the agent of sporotrichosis, an infection which is most commonly chronic and subcutaneous, or progressive and lymphocutaneous, but rarely also may manifest in an opportunistic respiratory or disseminated form. It affects humans and animals.

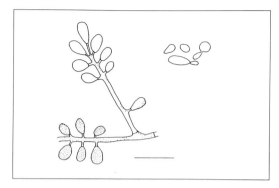

Figure 72.1 *Sporothrix schenckii. Filamentous form at 25°C and yeast form at 37°C.*

Ecology: cosmopolitan, isolated mainly from soil, from decomposing plant material, and living plants. Peat moss is a particularly well known source.

Dimorphic fungus

Colony appearance:

at 25°C:

- moderately rapid growth;
- texture glabrous, moist;
- color whitish to black on the surface and on the reverse.

at 37°C, on blood agar:

- moderately rapid growth;
- texture creamy
- color cream to beige.

Microscopic appearance:

at 25°C:

- hyphae septate, hyaline;
- conidiophores little differentiated from vegetative hyphae;
- conidia hyaline to brown, ovoid, thin-walled, grouped in rosettes at the tips of the conidiophores;
- brown conidia, ovoid or sometimes triangular, thick-walled, attached directly to the sides of hyphae.

at 37°C, on blood agar:

- yeasts ovoid or elongate, producing one or several buds.

Remarks: *S. schenckii* is distinguished by its greyish to black colonies on potato glucose agar, its hyaline conidia disposed in rosettes on denticles at the tips of conidiophores, and its brown, thick-walled conidia attached along the hyphae. In addition, it converts to a yeast phase at 37°C on rich media. Other, nonpathogenic *Sporothrix* species may in some cases convert to a yeast phase at 37°C, but do not produce brown, thick-walled conidia around the hyphae.

192

Ophiostoma stenoceras, a normally nonpathogenic species isolated occasionally in the clinical laboratory, possesses a *Sporothrix* state and produces its characteristic long-necked perithecia after 2-3 weeks of incubation.

Bibliography:

Dixon et al., 1991
Kwon-Chung, Bennett, 1992
Rippon, 1988

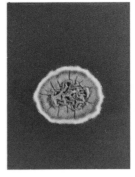
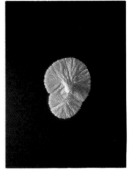

Figure 72.2   A, Filamentous form on Sabouraud glucose agar, 25°C, 7 days. B, Yeast form on brain-heart infusion agar, 37°C, 7 days.

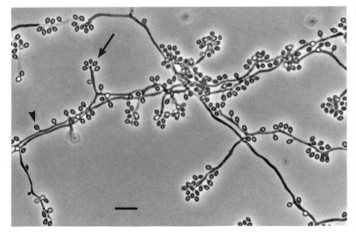
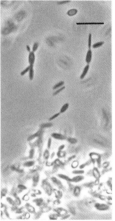

Figure 72.3   *Sporothrix schenckii.* A, Hyaline conidia in rosettes↑; brown, thick-walled conidia▲ formed along the hyphae. B, Yeasts formed at 37°C.

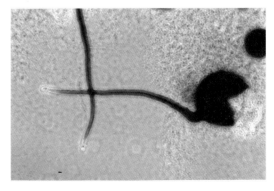

Figure 72.4   *Ophiostoma stenoceras.* Long-necked perithecia.

Sporotrichum Link ex Gray, 1821

Pathogenicity: commonly considered nonpathogenic. A few cases of repeated isolation of *Sporotrichum pruinosum* from respiratory secretions are suggestive of a bronchopulmonary colonization.

Ecology: cosmopolitan, isolated from decaying wood and from soil. These species are the anamorphs of basidiomycetous fungi which are important agents of wood decay.

Colony appearance:
- growth rapid to very rapid;
- texture powdery to lightly cottony;
- color white, rosy beige or orange.

Microscopic appearance:
- hyphae septate, with clamp connections absent or rare;
- conidiophores in the form of long, branched stalks;
- aleurioconidia unicellular, ellipsoidal to ovoid, truncate at the base, thick-walled, smooth, often terminal;
- arthroconidia often numerous, produced in dense clusters;
- chlamydospores spherical, sometimes measuring up to 60 um in diameter, always present at 25°C.

Remarks: unlike *Sporothrix*, *Sporotrichum* produces aleurioconidia with truncate bases and does not convert to a yeast phase at 37°C on rich media. It is distinguished from *Chrysosporium* by its numerous arthroconidia formed in chains which break up rapidly and form masses of loose conidia. *Chrysosporium* tends to have persistent chains of arthroconidia or, in some species, few or no arthroconidia. Also, *Sporotrichum* is distinguished by its large, thick-walled chlamydospores which, although similar in appearance to the adiaspores of *Emmonsia parva*, are not only formed at 37°C but also at 25°C. *Sporotrichum* species are normally inhibited by cycloheximide, while *Sporothrix* and *Chrysosporium* species tend not to be.

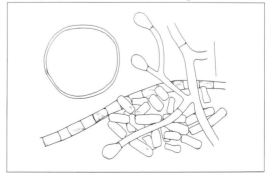

Figure 73.1   *Sporotrichum pruinosum.*

Bibliography:
Khan, Randhawa, Kowshik,
  Gaur, de Vries, 1988
McGinnis, 1980
Stalpers, 1984

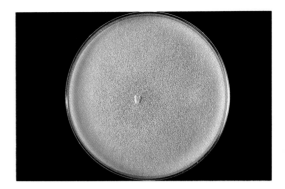

Figure 73.2 *Sporotrichum pruinosum.*
Potato glucose agar,
25°C, 7 days.

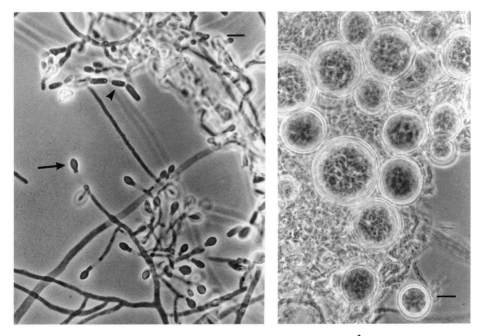

Figure 73.3 *Sporotrichum pruinosum.* A, Terminal conidia↑ formed on a
  long and frequently branched conidiophore; arthroconidia▲.
  B, Chlamydospores at 25°C.

195

Stachybotrys Corda, 1837

Pathogenicity: no cases of human or animal infection have been recorded. In humans, symptoms are noted following inhalation or percutaneous absorption of toxins elaborated by *Stachybotrys chartarum* (= *S. alternans*, = *S. atra*). Several cases of fatal intoxication have been noted in farm animals which have eaten feed contaminated by this fungus.

Ecology: cosmopolitan, saprobes commonly isolated from decaying plant material and soil. Prominent indoor habitats include water-damaged wallpapers and jute carpet backing along with their associated glues, plus moist debris in ducts and damp papers and books.

Colony appearance:
- growth moderately rapid;
- texture powdery;
- color white, pink, orange or black on the surface; reverse pale, orange, pink or black.

Microscopic appearance:
- hyphae septate, hyaline;
- conidiophores hyaline or pigmented, simple or branched, with smooth or rough walls;
- phialides hyaline or brown, ellipsoidal, formed in groups of 3 to 10 at the tips of the conidiophores;
- conidia black, unicellular, ellipsoidal, smooth to rough-walled, borne in slimy masses at the apices of the phialides.

Remarks: *S. chartarum* produces colonies in which both surface and reverse are black. *Stachybotrys* differs from *Memnoniella* by not producing conidia in chains. Both these genera are seldom isolated in the clinical laboratory.

Bibliography:

Domsch, Gams, Anderson, 1980
McGinnis, 1980

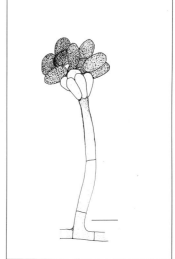

Figure 74.1   *Stachy-botrys chartarum.*

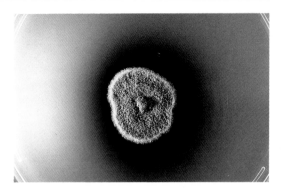

Figure 74.2 *Stachybotrys chartarum.*
Potato glucose agar,
25°C, 7 days.

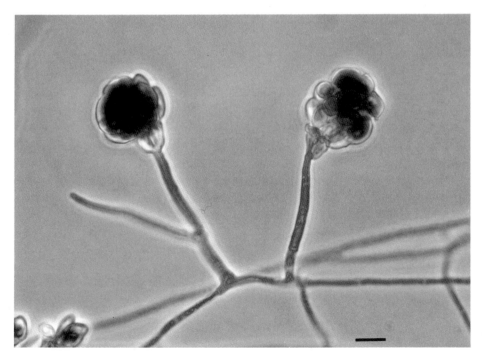

Figure 74.3 *Stachybotrys chartarum.* Black conidia formed on phialides
clustered at the apex of a conidiophore.

Syncephalastrum Schröter, 1886

Pathogenicity: no cases of infection have been reported in humans or animals.

Ecology: primarily present in tropical or subtropical regions, where they are saprobes commonly isolated from animal dung and soil.

Colony appearance:
- very rapid growth;
- texture wooly;
- color pale grey or dark grey on the surface; reverse pale.

Microscopic appearance:
- hyphae broad, with no or few septa;
- sporangiophores often branched, terminating in a vesicle;
- sporangia finger-shaped (merosporangia), formed around the vesicle;
- sporangiospores round, formed in a linear series in the interior of the merosporangia;
- rhizoids usually present.

Remarks: *Syncephalastrum* is classified within the order Mucorales. It produces sporangiophores terminating in a vesicle upon which merosporangia are fixed. It is necessary to avoid confusing these structures with *Aspergillus* heads.

Bibliography:
Domsch, Gams, Anderson, 1980
McGinnis, 1980

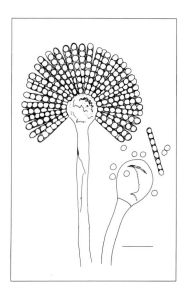

Figure 75.1   *Syncephalastrum* sp.

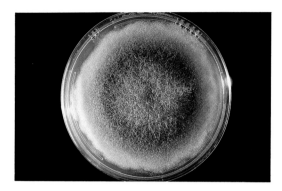

Figure 75.2 Potato glucose agar,
25°C, 7 days.

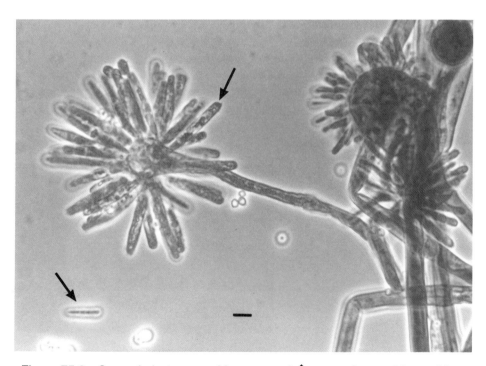

Figure 75.3 Syncephalastrum sp. Merosporangia↑ arranged around the vesicle
at the apex of a sporangiophore; detached merosporangium↑.

Trichoderma Persoon, 1801

Pathogenicity: usually considered nonpathogenic. Nonetheless, *Trichoderma viride* has been reported from a case of infection of a pulmonary cavity, as well as from a case of peritonitis in a dialysis patient and a case of perihepatic infection in a liver transplant patient.

Ecology: cosmopolitan, saprobes commonly isolated from soil and from wood.

Colony appearance:
- very rapid growth;
- texture wooly;
- color white, with scattered greenish tufts, sometimes arranged in concentric rings; reverse pale or yellowish.

Microscopic appearance:
- hyphae septate, hyaline;
- conidiophores hyaline, branched;
- phialides hyaline, inflated at the base, solitary or in clusters, attached at right angles on the conidiophores;
- conidia round or ellipsoidal, smooth-walled or rough, often green, in sticky heads at the tips of the phialides.

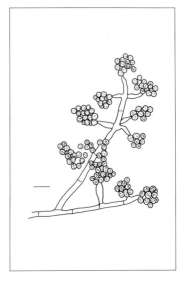

Figure 76.1   *Trichoderma* sp.

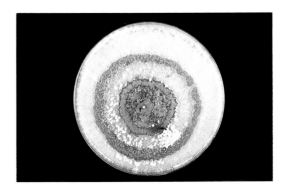

Figure 76.2   Potato glucose agar, 25°C, 7 days.

Remarks: *Trichoderma* species are contaminants occasionally encountered in the clinical laboratory. They are recognized by their wooly white colonies with scattered green tufts, their conidiophores and phialides in a pyramidal network, and their green conidia grouped in sticky heads. A few species with white conidia exist, but are very rarely seen in the clinical laboratory.

Bibliography:
Domsch, Gams, Anderson, 1980
Kwon-Chung, Bennett, 1992
McGinnis, 1980

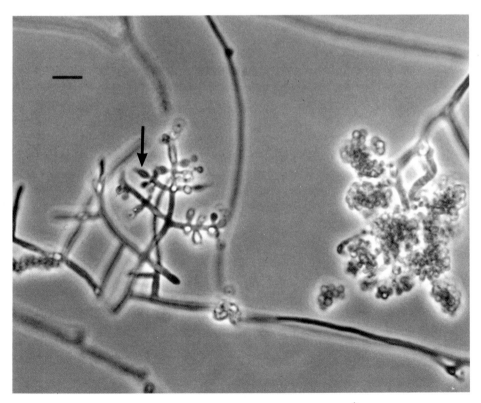

Figure 76.3   *Trichoderma* sp. Conidiophore and phialides[↑] arranged in a pyramidal network.

Trichophyton   Malmsten, 1845

Pathogenicity: the genus *Trichophyton* includes about 22 species of which 11 are commonly associated with tinea of the scalp, the nails, and the skin in humans. Only 4 species are frequently isolated from animals.

Ecology: includes anthropophilic, zoophilic and geophilic species. Certain *Trichophyton* species are cosmopolitan, while others have a limited geographic distribution.

Colony appearance:
- growth slow to moderately rapid;
- texture glabrous to downy;
- color white, yellowish, beige, or red violet on the surface; reverse pale, yellowish, brown or red brown.

Microscopic appearance:
- hyphae septate, hyaline;
- conidiophores little differentiated from vegetative hyphae;
- microconidia (microaleurioconidia) unicellular, round, pyriform, or club-shaped, solitary or in grape-like clusters.
- macroconidia (macroaleurioconidia) pluricellular, cylindrical, club-shaped, or cigar shaped, smooth-walled, often absent;
- arthroconidia and chlamydospores sometimes present;
- several species are typically sterile, but may be induced to form conidia on appropriate media.

Remarks: from a taxonomic point of view, *Trichophyton* is distinguished from *Microsporum* by its macroconidia with smooth walls. Notwithstanding this, for the identification of most species it is especially important to examine the morphology of the microconidia. In the species which are normally sterile in culture, the appearance of the colony, certain physiological tests, and sometimes the type of lesion will prove useful in identification.

Bibliography:
Kwon-Chung, Bennett, 1992
Rebell, Taplin, 1970
Rippon, 1988
Weitzman, Kane, 1991

Table IV. *Trichophyton*: characteristics of selected species.

Species	Colony			Macroconidia	Macroconidia	Hair perforation	Urease	Growth factor requirements
	Growth	Texture	Color (surface/reverse)					
T. ajelloi	moderately rapid	powdery, velvety	beige, orange / yellowish, blue black	fusiform, thick walled, numerous	pyriform, absent or rare	+	+	none
T. concentricum	very slow	glabrous, waxy	white, brown / white, brown	absent	absent	–	?	none or thiamine
T. equinum var. equinum	moderately rapid	downy	white, yellowish / yellow, red brown	club-shaped, absent or rare	pyriform, numerous	– (+)	+	nicotinic acid
T. megninii	moderately rapid	downy	pale pink / red	cylindrical, absent or rare	pyriform, club-shaped, numerous	–	+	histidine
T. mentagrophytes	moderately rapid	velvety, powdery	white / yellowish, brown, red brown	club-shaped, absent or ± numerous	pyriform, round, numerous or rare	+	+	none
T. rubrum	slow to moderately rapid	downy, powdery	white, pale pink / red, yellowish, brown	cylindrical, absent or ± numerous	club-shaped, pyriform, ± numerous	–	–	none
T. schoenleinii	very slow	glabrous	cream / cream	absent	absent	–	?	none
T. soudanense	slow	felty	yellowish, rusty / yellowish, rusty	absent	pyriform, ovoid, rare or absent	–	–	none (?)
T. terrestre	moderately rapid	powdery	cream, yellowish / yellowish	cylindrical, ± numerous	club-shaped, numerous	+	+	none
T. tonsurans	slow	powdery, downy	white, yellow, brown / brown, red brown	club-shaped, sinuous, absent or rare	club-shaped, balloon, numerous	– (+)	+	thiamine
T. verrucosum	very slow	glabrous	white, yellow / white, yellow	"rat tail", absent or rare	club-shaped, absent or rare	–	–	thiamine, inositol ±
T. violaceum	very slow	glabrous	red, violet / red, violet	absent	absent or rare	–	–	thiamine
T. yaoundei	very slow	glabrous	brown, cream / brown diffusible	absent	absent	–	?	none

Trichophyton ajelloi   (Vanbreuseghem) Ajello, 1968

Pathogenicity: normally considered nonpathogenic; the few cases of infection reported in humans and animals remain dubious.

Ecology: cosmopolitan, principally recovered from soil.

Colony appearance:
- moderately rapid growth;
- texture powdery to velvety;
- color beige to orange on the surface; reverse yellowish sometimes with a blue-black pigment diffusing into the medium.

Microscopic appearance:
- microconidia pyriform, often rare or absent;
- macroconidia numerous, multiseptate, long, cylindrical to fusiform, with a thick, smooth wall.

Physiological tests:
- urease: positive
- hair perforation: positive
- growth factor requirements: none

Remarks: *T. ajelloi* produces orange to beige colonies with a blue-black pigment diffusing into the medium in the reverse. Typically, its macroconidia are numerous, long and spindle- shaped; in contrast to the macroconidia of *Microsporum vanbreuseghemii*, their wall is smooth rather than rough.

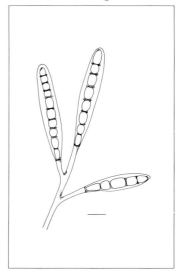

Figure 77.1   *Trichophyton ajelloi.*

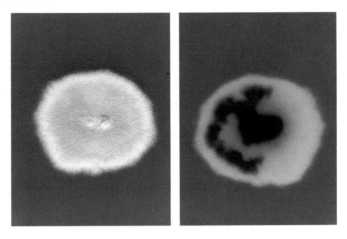

Figure 77.2 Sabouraud glucose agar,
25°C, 7 days (surface/reverse).

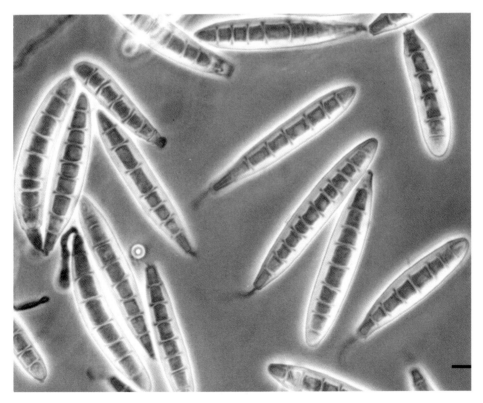

Figure 77.3 *Trichophyton ajelloi.* Macroconidia with smooth, thick walls.

Trichophyton concentricum Blanchard, 1896

Pathogenicity: agent of a dermatophytosis of the glabrous skin characterized by the formation of squamae in concentric and polycyclic rings that often cover the entire body.

Ecology: an anthropophilic dermatophyte found specifically in certain peoples from Oceania, Southeast Asia, Central America, and South America.

Colony appearance:
- very slow growth;
- texture glabrous, sometimes lightly downy;
- color white becoming cream, amber or brown on the surface; reverse white, pink or brown.

Microscopic appearance:
- hyphae septate, irregular, sometimes in favic chandeliers;
- macroconidia absent;
- microconidia absent.

Physiological tests:
- growth factor requirements: 50% of isolates stimulated by thiamine.

Remarks: *T. concentricum* is an anthropophilic dermatophyte with a restricted geographic distribution. It specifically attacks certain populations of humans. Its sterile colonies may sometimes be confused with those of *Trichophyton schoenleinii* and *Trichophyton verrucosum*. The clinical description of the infection in combination with information on the ethnic and geographic origin of the patient may be useful in diagnosis.

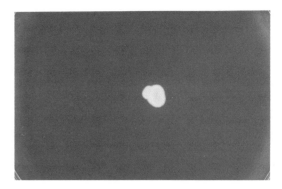

Figure 78.1   Sabouraud glucose agar,
25°C, 7 days.

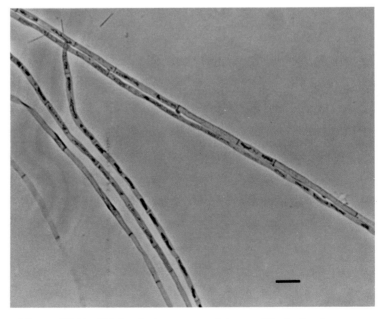

Figure 78.2   *Trichophyton concentricum*. Sterile hyphae.

Trichophyton equinum

(Matruchot et Dassonville) Gedoelst, 1902

Pathogenicity: a common cause of dermatophytosis in the horse, only rarely infecting humans.

Ecology: a zoophilic dermatophyte found principally in association with the horse. It exists in two varieties: *T. equinum* var. *equinum*, with a worldwide distribution, and *T. equinum* var. *autotrophicum*, found only in Australia and New Zealand.

Colony appearance:
- moderately rapid growth;
- texture downy;
- color cream to pale yellow on the surface; reverse deep yellow becoming red-brown.

Microscopic appearance:
- microconidia pyriform, formed along the hyphae, rarely in rebranching clusters;
- macroconidia very rare, fusiform to club-shaped, similar to those of *Trichophyton mentagrophytes*.

Physiological tests:
- urease: positive
- hair perforation: negative (sometimes positive)
- growth factor requirements: requirement for nicotinic acid (var. *equinum*) or, no requirements (var. *autotrophicum*)
- BCP-milk solids-glucose: alkalinization

Remarks: *T. equinum* produces white colonies with a deep yellow to red-brown reverse, and has pyriform microconidia formed along otherwise ordinary-looking hyphae. Unlike *T. mentagrophytes*, *T. equinum* var. *equinum*, the most widely distributed variety, requires a supply of nicotinic acid for growth.

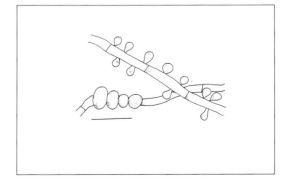

Figure 79.1   *Trichophyton equinum.*

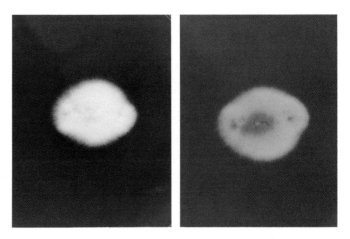

Figure 79.2   Sabouraud glucose agar,
25°C, 7 days (surface/reverse).

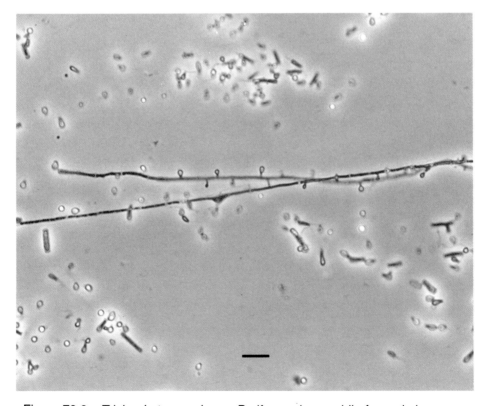

Figure 79.3   *Trichophyton equinum.* Pyriform microconidia formed along
hyphae.

Trichophyton megninii   Blanchard, 1896

Pathogenicity: an agent of tinea of the glabrous skin, the scalp and the beard. No cases of animal infection have been reported.

Ecology: an anthropophilic dermatophyte with geographic distribution restricted to parts of Europe (especially Portugal and Italy) and certain regions of Africa.

Colony appearance:
- moderately rapid growth;
- texture felty to downy;
- color pale pink on the surface; reverse deep red.

Microscopic appearance:
- microconidia pyriform or club-shaped;
- macroconidia rare, pencil-shaped or cigar-shaped, similar to those of *Trichophyton rubrum*

Physiological tests:
- urease: positive (urea broth)
- hair perforation: negative
- growth factor requirements: requires histidine
- BCP-milk solids-glucose: alkalinization

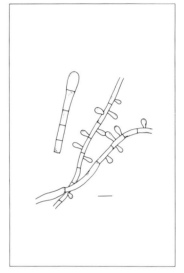

Figure 80.1   *Trichophyton megninii.*

Remarks: *T. megninii* is distinguished from *T. rubrum* and *T. mentagrophytes* by its requirement for histidine. It also differs from *T. rubrum* by producing urease; however, to ensure accuracy in this case, it is essential to perform this test in liquid medium (urea-indole broth), rather than on Christensen urea agar, which may give negative results in the recommended 7 days of incubation. It is also necessary to ensure that *T. rubrum* colonies are completely uncontaminated by urease positive bacteria of the normal skin flora; these are usually not eliminated by medium antibacterials and are seldom visible on macroscopic examination of colonies. *T. megninii*, unlike *T. mentagrophytes*, does not perforate hair *in vitro*.

Bibliography:
Sequeira, Cabrita, de Vroey, Wytack-Raes, 1991

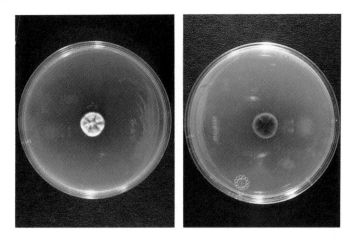

Figure 80.2   Sabouraud glucose agar,
25°C, 7 days (surface/reverse).

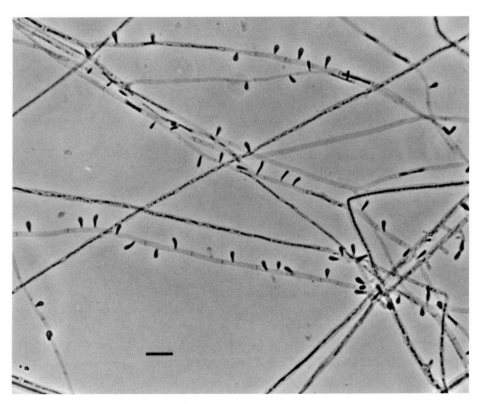

Figure 80.3   *Trichophyton megninii*.   Club-shaped microconidia.

Trichophyton mentagrophytes (Robin) Blanchard, 1896

Pathogenicity: anthropophilic isolates, often referred to as *T. mentagrophytes* var. *interdigitale*, are a frequent cause of chronic infection of the feet, the nails and the groin. Zoophilic isolates such as *T. mentagrophytes* var. *mentagrophytes*, when infecting humans, are more often associated with inflammatory lesions of the scalp, the glabrous skin, the nails, and the beard region. Other varieties exist, but are only occasionally isolated in humans.

Ecology: cosmopolitan dermatophytes, anthropophilic or zoophilic. Certain small mammals (rodents, hedgehogs, rabbits) appear to be the principal reservoirs of the zoophilic varieties in nature, although many other species of animals may also be infected.

Colony appearance:
- moderately rapid growth;
- texture downy to powdery (anthropophilic isolates) or granular (zoophilic isolates);
- color white to cream on the surface; reverse yellowish, brown or red brown.

Microscopic appearance:
- spiral hyphae often present;
- microconidia unicellular, round to pyriform, in closely rebranched clusters or along otherwise undifferentiated hyphae, usually numerous, sometimes rare in anthropophilic isolates;
- macroconidia multiseptate, mostly club-shaped, with thin, smooth walls, solitary, often absent.

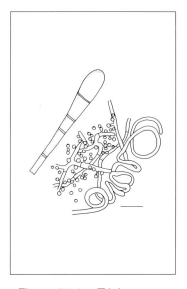

Figure 81.1 *Tricho-phyton mentagro-phytes.*

Physiological tests:
- urease: positive
- hair perforation: positive
- growth factor requirements: none
- BCP-milk solids-glucose: alkalinization and profuse growth

Remarks: *T. mentagrophytes* is usually distinguished from *Trichophyton rubrum* by its rounded conidia borne in dense clusters, its spiral hyphae and its colonies with brownish reverse pigmentation. These characters, however, are sometimes absent in anthropophilic isolates. Positive reactions in the urease and hair perforation tests, as well as the alkalinization seen on BCP-milk solids-glucose agar, are more stable criteria. Unlike *Microsporum persicolor*, *T. mentagrophytes* grows abundantly at 37°C and produces an alkaline reaction on BCP-milk solids- glucose agar.

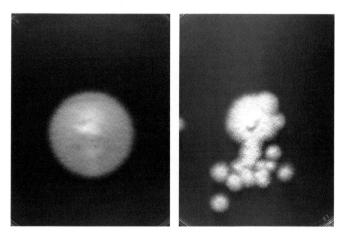

Figure 81.2   Sabouraud glucose agar, 25°C, 7 days.
Downy colony and powdery colony.

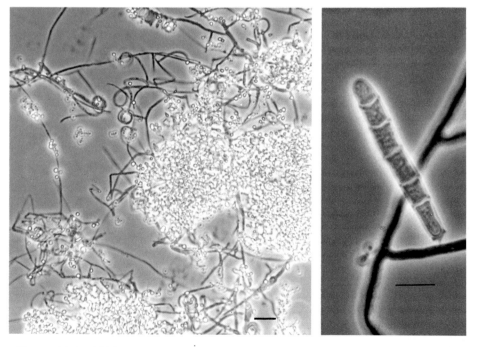

Figure 81.3   *Trichophyton mentagrophytes.* A, Round microconidia on clustered branches and spiral hyphae. B, Club-shaped macroconidium.

Trichophyton rubrum   (Castellani) Sabouraud, 1911

Pathogenicity: a common cause of tinea of the groin, the glabrous skin, the feet, the hands and the nails; the scalp is very rarely infected. Animals are very rarely infected.

Ecology: the most widespread of the anthropophilic dermatophytes.

Colony appearance:
- growth slow to moderately rapid;
- texture downy, sometimes powdery;
- color white to pale pink on the surface; reverse typically wine red, sometimes brown, violet, yellow or even uncolored.

Microscopic appearance:
- microconidia numerous to rare, unicellular, club-shaped to pyriform, solitary along hyphae or sometimes in clusters;
- macroconidia multiseptate, pencil-shaped or cigar-shaped, often absent.

Physiological tests:
- urease: negative
- hair perforation: negative
- growth factor requirements: none
- BCP-milk solids-glucose: no change in pH, restricted growth
- potato glucose agar or cornmeal glucose agar favor the production of red pigment on the reverse of the majority of isolates which remain unpigmented on Sabouraud glucose agar.

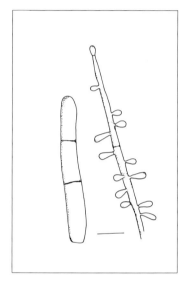

Figure 82.1   *Trichophyton rubrum.*

Remarks: in contrast to *Trichophyton mentagrophytes, T. rubrum* produces microconidia which are more club-shaped than round, and is urease negative, fails to perforate hair *in vitro*, and does not change the pH of BCP-milk solids-glucose agar within 7 days. *Trichophyton raubitschekii* is a species narrowly delineated from *T. rubrum*: it usually originates from Asia, Africa, or the Mediterranean, and is distinguished by its numerous cigar-shaped macroconidia, its often round microconidia, and its positive urease test. Unlike *T. megninii, T. rubrum* does not require a supply of histidine for growth.

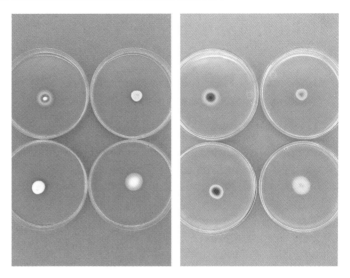

Figure 82.2   *Trichophyton rubrum*. Sabouraud
glucose, 25°C, 7 days. Various types
of colonies (surface/reverse).

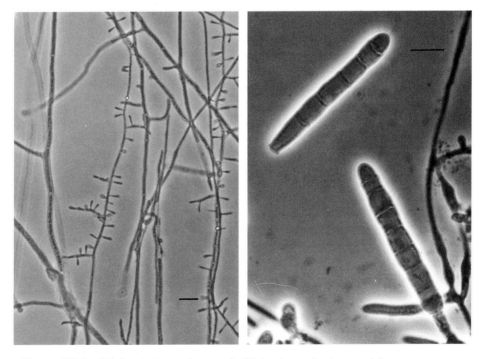

Figure 82.3   *Trichophyton rubrum*. A, Club-shaped microconidia.
B, Cigar-shaped macroconidia.

Trichophyton schoenleinii

(Lebert) Langeron et Milochevitch, 1930

Pathogenicity: agent of favus (tinea favosa) of the scalp, an infection characterized by the presence of scutula, that is, crusts or cupules composed of an accumulation of hyphae and skin debris. Infection of animals is rare.

Ecology: an anthropophilic dermatophyte mainly isolated in certain regions of Eurasia and Africa. It has previously been found in certain small endemic areas in the Americas, but has likely now been extirpated from most or all of them.

Colony appearance:
- very slow growth;
- texture glabrous to waxy, becoming velvety on subculture;
- color cream on the surface and on the reverse.

Microscopic appearance:
- hyphae in the form of "favic chandeliers", or with "nail head" tips often present in the submerged mycelium;
- microconidia typically absent;
- macroconidia typically absent.

Physiological tests:
- urease: variable
- hair perforation: negative
- growth factor requirements: none
- BCP-milk solids-glucose: alkalinization

Remarks: *T. schoenleinii* produces pallid, folded, upraised, glabrous or waxy colonies. In microscopic examination, "favic chandeliers" are typically present. In contrast to *Trichophyton verrucosum*, it has no nutritional requirement for thiamine or inositol and grows as well at 25°C as at 37°C.

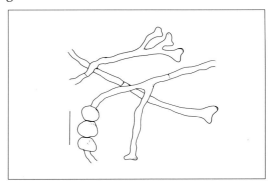

Figure 83.1   *Trichophyton schoenleinii.*

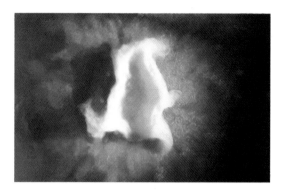

Figure 83.2   Sabouraud glucose agar,
25°C, 21 days.

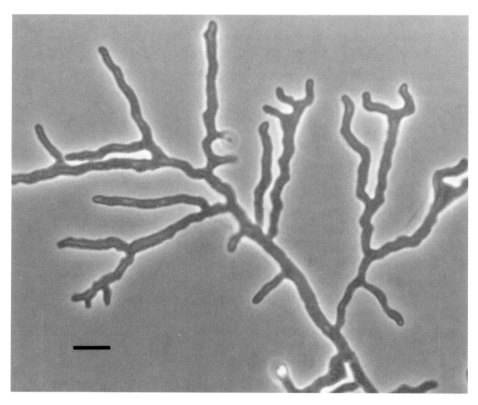

Figure 83.3   *Trichophyton schoenleinii.* Favic chandeliers.

217

Trichophyton soudanense Joyeux, 1912

Pathogenicity: a frequent cause of inflammatory tinea of the scalp in Africa. Animal infection is very rare.

Ecology: an anthropophilic dermatophyte with endemic zones limited to certain regions of Africa.

Colony appearance:
- growth slow to moderately rapid;
- texture glabrous to felty, with a filamentous fringe around the colony;
- color pale yellow to rusty, sometimes red purple; surface and reverse similar.

Microscopic appearance:
- hyphae with reflexive branching typically present;
- microconidia more or less rare, pyriform to ovoid, solitary or in groups;
- macroconidia usually absent.

Physiological tests:
- urease: usually negative
- hair perforation: negative
- growth factor requirements: none, or, commonly, uncharacterized requirements which cause many isolates subcultured onto *Trichophyton* agars to show no signs of growth until after at least 3 weeks of incubation, with some isolates appearing completely incapable of growth
- Lowenstein-Jensen: dark brown to black colonies
- BCP-milk solids-glucose: alkalization, small peripheral zone of hydrolytic clearing

Remarks: *T. soudanense* produces straw- to rust-colored colonies surrounded by a fringe of hyphae. In the microscope, bundles of hyphae with reflexive branching, that is, nearby branches pointing in opposing directions, are typically observed, especially in the surface hyphae of the radial fringe. Unlike *Microsporum ferrugineum*, *T. soudanense* takes on a deep brown coloration on Lowenstein-Jensen medium, and causes alkalinization of BCP-milk solids-glucose agar.

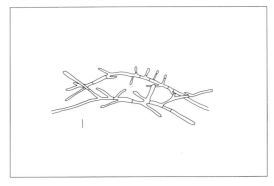

Figure 84.1   *Trichophyton soudanense.*

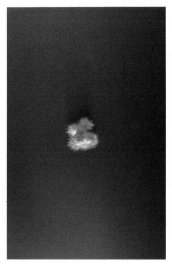 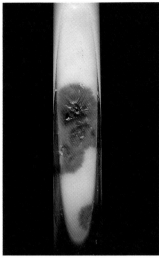

Figure 84.2   A, Sabouraud glucose agar,
              25°C, 7 days (surface/reverse).
              B, Lowenstein-Jensen agar,
              25°C, 14 days.

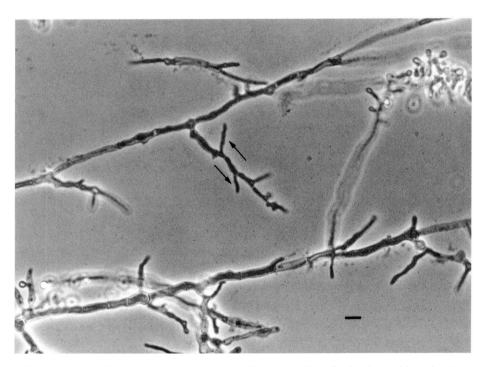

Figure 84.3   *Trichophyton soudanense*. Hyphae with reflexive branching, that is,
              nearby branches pointing in opposing directions↑.

Trichophyton terrestre

Durie et Frey, 1957

Pathogenicity: no cases of infection demonstrated in humans or animals.

Ecology: cosmopolitan, geophilic.   Often isolated from the fur of small mammals or from alkaline and arid soils.

Colony appearance:
- moderately rapid growth at 25°C; no growth at 37°C;
- texture powdery to downy;
- color cream to pale yellow on the surface; reverse yellowish, sometimes red.

Microscopic appearance:
- microconidia pyriform to club-shaped, often elongate, often borne on pedicels;
- macroconidia cylindrical, with smooth, thin walls, 2-6 cells long.

Physiological tests:
- urease: positive
- hair perforation: positive
- growth factor requirements: none
- BCP-milk solids-glucose: alkalinization, profuse growth

Remarks: isolates of *T. terrestre* produce elongate microconidia, often on pedicels, as well as cylindrical macroconidia made up of 2-6 cells. Unlike *T. mentagrophytes*, *T. terrestre* does not grow at 37°C.

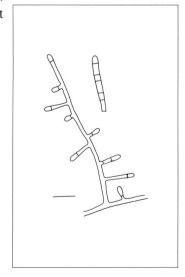

Figure 85.1   *Trichophyton terrestre.*

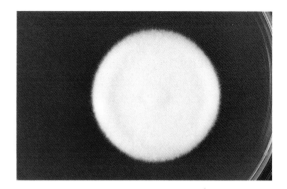

Figure 85.2   Sabouraud glucose agar,
25°C, 7 days.

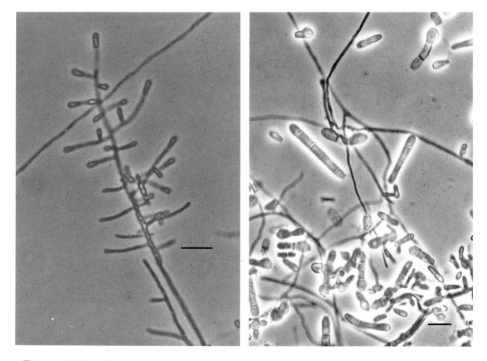

Figure 85.3   *Trichophyton terrestre.* A, Pedicellate microconidia.
B, Macroconidia.

Trichophyton tonsurans   Malmsten, 1845

Pathogenicity: a dermatophyte principally responsible for infections of the scalp and sometimes of the glabrous skin or the nails. Rarely isolated from animals.

Ecology: cosmopolitan, anthropophilic. Particularly common in Mexico, in the other countries of Latin America, and in large cities in the United States.

Colony appearance:
- slow growth;
- texture variable, suede-like, sometimes powdery or velvety;
- color white, beige, pale yellow, sulfur yellow, or brown on the surface; reverse yellow, dark brown, or red-brown.

Microscopic appearance:
- microconidia numerous, of varying shapes and sizes (pyriform, club-shaped, or balloon shaped);
- macroconidia rare, sinuous, with thin, smooth walls.

Physiological tests:
- urease: positive
- hair perforation: negative (sometimes positive)
- growth factor requirements: growth stimulated by thiamine
- BCP-milk solids-glucose: most isolates produce alkalinization of the medium

Remarks: *T. tonsurans* is distinguished from *T. mentagrophytes* by its microconidia of diverse shapes and sizes, and by the stimulating effect of thiamine on its growth. In contrast to *Trichophyton soudanense*, this cosmopolitan dermatophyte produces abundant conidia and shows a clear thiamine response.

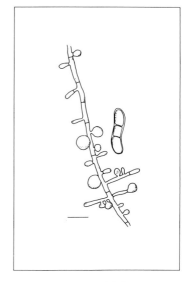

Figure 86.1   *Trichophyton tonsurans.*

222

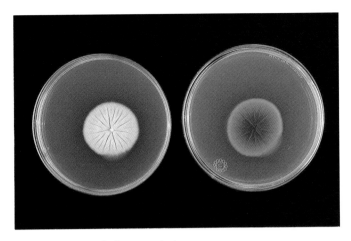

Figure 86.2   Sabouraud glucose agar,
25°C, 7 days (surface/reverse).

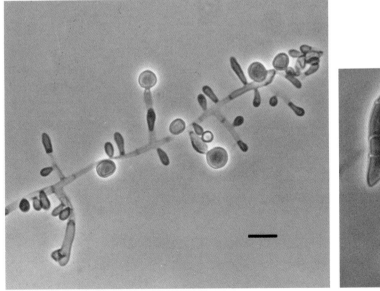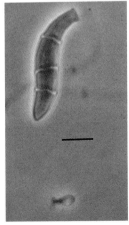

Figure 86.3   *Trichophyton tonsurans.* A, Microconidia of variable
morphology. B, Sinuous macroconidium.

223

Trichophyton verrucosum   Bodin, 1902

Pathogenicity: a frequent cause of dermatophytosis of cattle and other farm animals. When contracted from an infected animal, it most commonly provokes a strongly inflammatory infection in humans. This infection typically occurs in the scalp, the beard region, or the glabrous skin.

Ecology: cosmopolitan, a zoophilic dermatophyte frequently isolated from cattle and horses.

Colony appearance:
- very slow growth; more rapid at 37°C than at 25°C;
- texture glabrous, sometimes lightly downy;
- color white, sometimes yellow or greyish on the surface; reverse without any characteristic pigment.

Microscopic appearance:
- microconidia club-shaped, often absent;
- macroconidia "rat tail" shaped, very rare;
- chlamydospores in chains typically present.

Physiological tests:
- urease: negative
- hair perforation: negative
- growth factor requirements: thiamine required, and also often inositol
- BCP-milk solids-glucose: no pH change, wide zone of hydrolytic clearing around the colonies

Remarks: *T. verrucosum* is distinguished by its small, glabrous, and pale colonies which develop more rapidly at 37°C than at 25°C. It typically produces chlamydospores in chains, often more numerous at 37°C. In contrast to *T. schoenleinii*, its growth is almost always dependent on thiamine and often also on inositol.

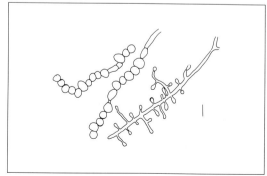

Figure 87.1   *Trichophyton verrucosum.*

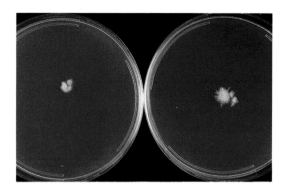

Figure 87.2   Sabouraud glucose agar,
7 days, 25° and 37°C.

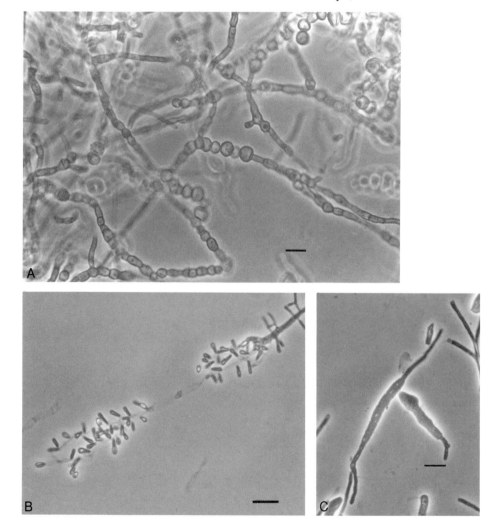

Figure 87.3   *Trichophyton verrucosum* . A, Chains of chlamydospores.
B, Microconidia. C, Rat-tail shaped macroconidia,
rarely present.

225

Trichophyton violaceum   Sabouraud in Bodin, 1902

Pathogenicity: primarily isolated from tinea of the scalp, though it is capable of infecting the glabrous skin, the nails, and the soles of the feet. Animals are rarely infected.

Ecology: an anthropophilic species mostly from north Africa and the Middle East, but also from parts of Europe. Some endemic foci exist in South America and Mexico.

Colony appearance:
- very slow growth;
- texture glabrous;
- color deep red to violet on surface and reverse.

Microscopic appearance:
- hyphae irregular in diameter;
- microconidia typically absent, sometimes present on media enriched with thiamine;
- macroconidia typically absent;
- chlamydospores often formed in age.

Physiological tests:
- urease: negative
- hair perforation: negative
- growth factor requirements: growth stimulated by thiamine

Remarks: *T. violaceum* produces small, glabrous, red to violet colonies. They are typically sterile and require thiamine for growth. They rapidly lose their color on subculture.

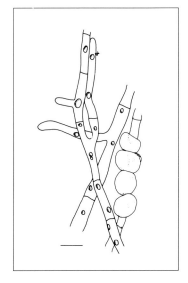

Figure 88.1   *Tricophyton violaceum.*

226

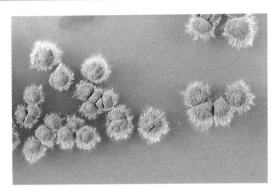

Figure 88.2   Sabouraud glucose agar,
25°C, 14 days.

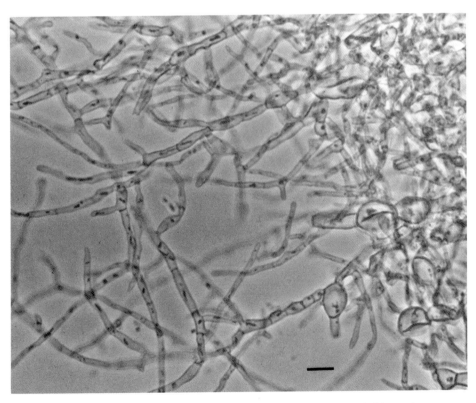

Figure 88.3   *Trichophyton violaceum*.   Deformed hyphae and chlamydospores.

227

Trichophyton yaoundei   Cochet et Doby-Dubois, nom. inval.

Pathogenicity: mainly associated with inflammatory tinea of the scalp. No cases have been reported in animals.

Ecology: an anthropophilic dermatophyte endemic to equatorial Africa, in particular Cameroons, Zaire, and Mozambique.

Colony appearance:
- very slow growth;
- texture glabrous;
- color cream becoming chocolate brown on the surface and on the reverse; a brown diffusible pigment is present within the medium in mature colonies.

Microscopic appearance:
- hyphae of irregular diameter; favic chandeliers sometimes present;
- microconidia pyriform, rare;
- macroconidia very rare;
- chlamydospores often present.

Physiological tests:
- hair perforation: negative
- growth factor requirements: none

Remarks: *T. yaoundei* is distinguished by its glabrous, cream-colored colonies, becoming chocolate brown with age and producing a brown diffusible pigment within the medium. The absence of nutrient requirements may aid the differentiation from *Trichophyton verrucosum*.

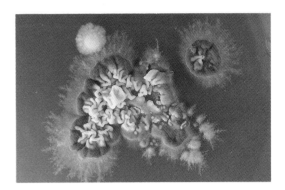

Figure 89.1 Sabouraud glucose agar, 25°C, 21 days.

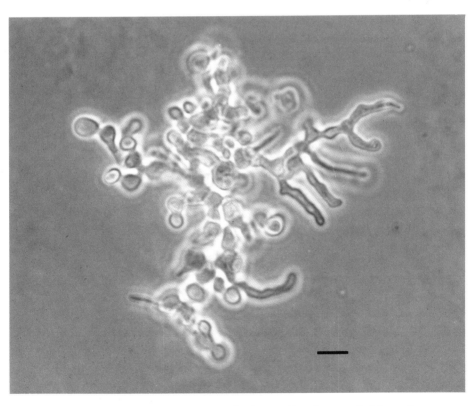

Figure 89.2 *Trichophyton yaoundei*. Deformed hyphae and chlamydospores.

229

Trichothecium   Link, 1809

Pathogenicity: no case of infection has been recorded in humans or animals.

Ecology: cosmopolitan, saprobes commonly isolated from decaying plant material. Several species are parasites of fleshy fungi.

Colony appearance:
- rapid growth;
- texture powdery;
- color white becoming pale pink on the surface; reverse pale.

Microscopic appearance:
- hyphae septate, hyaline;
- conidiophores unbranched;
- conidia two-celled, broadly club-shaped, overlapping in an imbricate, zigzag column at the tip of the conidiophore.

Remarks: *Trichothecium* produces powdery, pale pink colonies with broadly club-shaped, bicellular conidia. While the conidia of *Microsporum nanum* are solitary, those of *Trichothecium* cohere at the ends of the conidiophores in imbricate, zigzagging groups. Within these groups, individual conidia alternate in opposite directions as they stack up into a delicate column; new conidia are added at the bottom of the column. Additionally, *Trichothecium* differs from *M. nanum* in that it does not perforate hair *in vitro*, and is inhibited by the cycloheximide in Mycosel agar.

Bibliography:
Domsch, Gams, Anderson, 1980
McGinnis, 1980

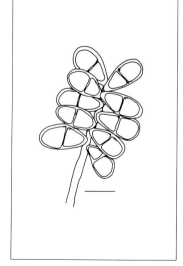

Figure 90.1   *Tricho-thecium* sp.

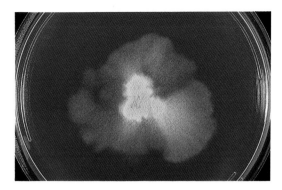

Figure 90.2   Potato glucose agar,
25°C, 7 days.

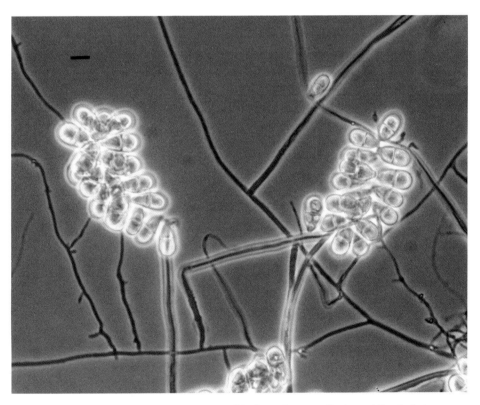

Figure 90.3   *Trichothecium roseum*. Chains of two-celled conidia, imbricate
in a zigzagging arrangement.

Tritirachium

Pathogenicity: no case of infection has been recorded in humans or animals.

Ecology: cosmopolitan, saprobes commonly isolated from decaying plant material.

Colony appearance:
- slow growth;
- texture downy;
- color yellowish, cinnamon or purple on the surface; reverse pale.

Microscopic appearance:
- hyphae septate, hyaline;
- conidiophores long and narrow;
- conidiogenous cells elongate, inflated at the base, tapering and terminating in a narrow zigzag structure, grouped in verticils around the conidiophore;
- conidia unicellular, round to ellipsoidal.

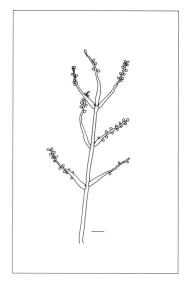

Figure 91.1   *Tritirachium sp.*

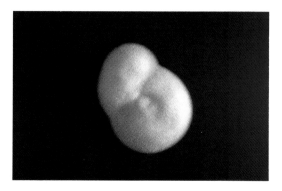

Figure 91.2   Potato glucose agar, 25°C, 7 days.

Remarks: *Tritirachium* is distinguished from *Beauveria* by its conidio-genous cells grouped in verticils around the conidiophores.

Bibliography:
Barron, 1968

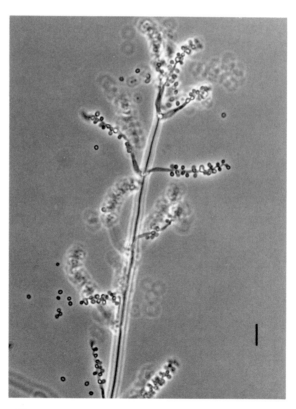

Figure 91.3   *Tritirachium* sp. Conidiogenous cells terminating in zigzagging structures, grouped in verticils around the conidiophore.

Ulocladium Preuss, 1851

Pathogenicity: no case of infection has been reported in humans or animals.

Ecology: cosmopolitan, saprobes of decaying plant material.

Colony appearance:
- moderately rapid growth;
- texture wooly to cottony;
- color olive brown to black on the surface and on the reverse.

Microscopic appearance:
- hyphae septate, brown;
- conidiophores brown, strongly geniculate;
- conidia (poroconidia) brown, muriform, obovoid to ellipsoidal, with smooth or rough walls, often produced singly, uncommonly in short chains.

Remarks: *Ulocladium* is distinguished from *Alternaria* by its strongly geniculate conidiophores, and its rather obovoid (egg- shaped, narrower at the base than at the apex) conidia formed singly in almost all species. When species are encountered which do produce short chains of conidia, these conidia may exhibit a short, tubular outgrowth at the point where the secondary conidium forms, but do not possess a tapered apex elongated into a beak as is found in many *Alternaria* conidia. Unlike *Curvularia*, *Bipolaris* and *Drechslera*, *Ulocladium* produces conidia which possess both longitudinal and transverse septa (muriform).

Bibliography:
Domsch, Gams, Anderson, 1980
McGinnis, 1980

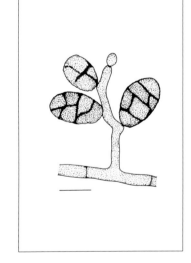

Figure 92.1   *Ulocladium* sp.

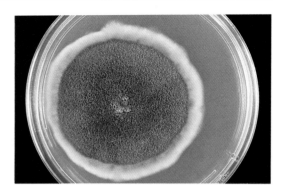

Figure 92.2   Potato glucose agar,
25°C, 7 days.

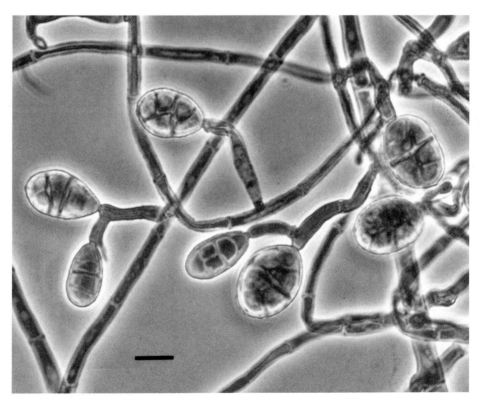

Figure 92.3   *Ulocladium* sp.   Geniculate conidiophore and muriform conidia.

Verticillium

Nees, 1817

Pathogenicity: normally considered nonpathogenic; some cases of keratitis have been indicated but remain dubious.

Ecology: cosmopolitan, isolated from soil and decaying plant material. Certain species are parasites of other fungi, plants, or arthropods.

Colony appearance:
- growth moderately rapid to rapid;
- texture velvety to wooly;
- color white, yellowish, pinkish brown or rarely green on the surface; reverse often with little pigment or brown.

Microscopic appearance:
- hyphae septate, hyaline;
- conidiophores hyaline, simple or branched;
- phialides hyaline, long and narrow, grouped in verticils around the conidiophore.
- conidia hyaline, unicellular, ovoid to pyriform, sometimes in sticky heads at the tips of phialides.

Remarks: *Verticillium* produces long, narrow phialides which, unlike those typical of *Acremonium*, are not solitary but are grouped in verticils around the conidiophore. Occasionally in the clinical laboratory, isolates of *Verticillium* are encountered which produce only solitary phialides. In general, these species produce colonies which grow more rapidly and are more wooly in texture than are *Acremonium* colonies. A detailed microscopic study of these isolates often allows the discovery of at least some phialides grouped in verticils.

Bibliography:
Domsch, Gams, Anderson, 1980
McGinnis, 1980

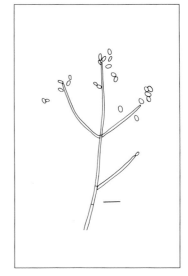

Figure 93.1   *Verticillium sp.*

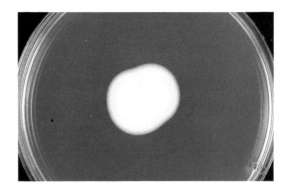

Figure 93.2   Potato glucose agar,
25°C, 7 days.

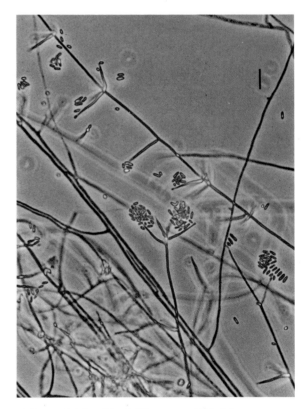

Figure 93.3   *Verticillium* sp. Phialides
arranged in verticils around
a conidiophore.

Wangiella dermatitidis McGinnis, 1977

Pathogenicity: *Wangiella dermatitidis* is an occasional agent of subcutaneous phaeohyphomycosis and sometimes also of disseminated infection in the immunocompromised patient. Primary infection is usually subsequent to the implantation of the fungus into the dermis, and the organism normally remains localized.

Ecology: cosmopolitan, a saprobe from soil and plants.

Colony appearance:
- slow growth;
- texture viscous becoming lightly velvety around the periphery;
- color black to olive black on the surface and on the reverse.

Microscopic appearance:
- hyphae septate, brown, often toruloid;
- conidiophores not or scarcely differentiated from vegetative hyphae;
- phialides brown, ellipsoidal, without collarettes, little differentiated;
- conidia pale brown, unicellular, oval;
- brown yeasts typically present.

Remarks: the genus *Wangiella* consists of only a single species, *W. dermatitidis*. This organism produces, in primary isolation, colonies of viscous to creamy texture composed of black budding yeasts. These cells eventually give rise to septate hyphae bearing rather undistinguished, ellipsoidal phialides, which produce oval conidia. In contrast to *Exophiala jeanselmei*, *W. dermatitidis* grows at 40°C and does not assimilate potassium nitrate.

Bibliography:
Dixon, Polak-Wyss, 1990
Kwon-Chung, Bennett, 1992
McGinnis, 1980

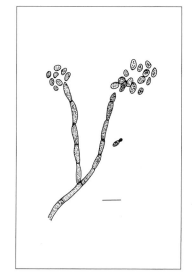

Figure 94.1 *Wangiella dermatitidis.*

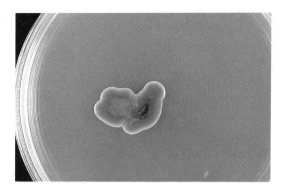

Figure 94.2   Potato glucose agar,
25°C, 7 days.

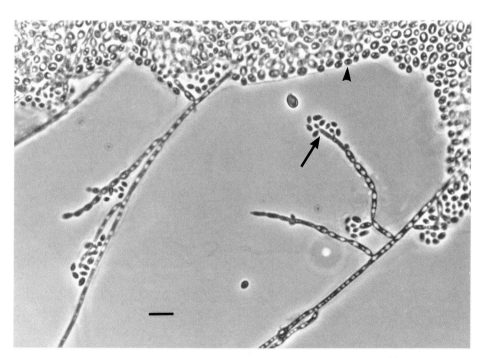

Figure 94.3   *Wangiella dermatitidis*. Conidiophores and phialides[↑] poorly
differentiated from vegetative hyphae; yeast cells▲.

Xylohypha

(Fries) Nason apud Deighton, 1960

Pathogenicity: normally nonpathogenic, with the exception of *Xylohypha bantiana* (= *Cladosporium bantianum*, = *Cladosporium trichoides* sensu Kwon-Chung), an agent of cerebral phaeohyphomycosis, and *Xylohypha emmonsii*, isolated in several cases of subcutaneous infection in humans and animals.

Ecology: cosmopolitan, saprobes from soil and decaying plant material. *X. bantiana* is often associated with trees in the family Cupressaceae, especially cedars and junipers. Most infections caused by this organism have been contracted in the southeastern United States.

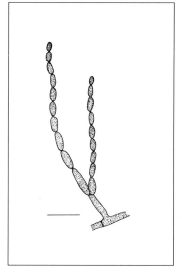

Figure 95.1 *Xylohypha bantiana.*

Colony appearance:
- moderately rapid growth;
- texture downy;
- color olive grey to black on surface and reverse.

Microscopic appearance:
- hyphae septate, brown;
- conidiophores brown, septate, not differentiated from vegetative hyphae;
- conidia unicellular, clear brown in color, ellipsoidal, in long (20 to 35 cells), infrequently branched chains, which are resistant to disarticulation.

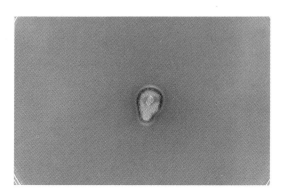

Figure 95.2 *Xylohypha bantiana.*
Potato glucose agar,
25°C, 7 days.

Remarks: it is not yet clearly established whether or not cerebral infections with *X. bantiana* are acquired via pulmonary exposure. Given that normal, immunocompetent hosts may be infected and that the disease is always fatal, the use of a biological safety cabinet is recommended as a safety precaution for workers manipulating cultures of this organism. *X. bantiana* and *X. emmonsii* are distinguished from nonpathogenic *Cladosporium* by the absence of distinct conidiophores and by their tolerance of temperatures above 37°C. *X. emmonsii* is distinguished from *X. bantiana* by its maximal growth temperature of 38°C rather than the 42-43°C maximum of the latter. Also, *X. emmonsii* typically has sigmoid conidia, in shorter chains than those of *X. bantiana*.

Bibliography:
McGinnis, Borelli, Padhye, Ajello, 1986
Padhye et al., 1988
Rippon, 1988

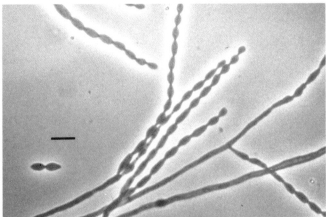

Figure 95.3   *Xylohypha bantiana*. Conidia in long, infrequently branched chains.

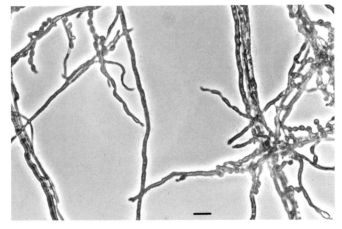

Figure 95.4   *Xylohypha emmonsii*. Sigmoid conidia[↑] in chain.

Methods

Identification of dermatophytes

Identification of dimorphic fungi

Miscellaneous

Culture on autoclaved rice grains

Objective
To aid the distinction of *Microsporum audouinii* from poorly pigmented or sterile isolates of *Microsporum canis*.

Principle
Unfortified white rice is not sufficiently rich to allow the growth of *M. audouinii*. It does, however, support good growth in *Microsporum canis*, and at the same time stimulates the production of yellow pigment and typical macroconidia.

Method
1)   Inoculate some grains of cooked, autoclaved rice with small pieces of inoculum from the colony.

2)   Incubate at 25°C for 7 days.

3)   Observe growth and pigment production.

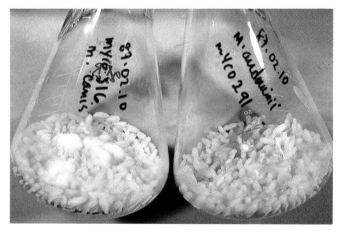

Figure 96.   Cultures of *Microsporum canis* (left) and *Microsporum audouinii* (right) on autoclaved rice grains.

244

Quality control

M. canis	rapid growth with yellow pigment and production of macroconidia.
M. audouinii	no growth or minimal growth with production of a brownish pigment in the rice.

Bibliography
Rebell, Taplin, 1970

Growth factor requirements

Objective
To confirm the identification of certain dermatophytes in the genus *Trichophyton*.

Principle
The *Trichophyton* agars are a series of seven media differing in ingredients. Agars #1 and #6 are basal media serving as controls, while the remaining media contain specifically added vitamins or amino acids. The requirement of a dermatophyte isolate for these molecules is seen in an enhancement of growth on the supplemented media, compared to slower, thinner growth on the corresponding basal control medium.

Method
1) Inoculate each *Trichophyton* agar with a small fragment around 1 mm in diameter from an actively growing colony on Sabouraud glucose agar. Ordinarily, media #1 and #4 (see composition in the section on culture media) are the most useful. When inoculating the media, it is necessary to take care not to transfer agar from the primary culture to the *Trichophyton* agars. The nutrient substances in Sabouraud glucose agar, if transferred, may alter the chemical composition of the *Trichophyton* agars and give rise to false results. Bacterial contamination may also invalidate the test results, since certain bacteria may synthesize the vitamin necessary for fungal growth.

2) Incubate at 25°C for a period of 14 days and perform a preliminary examination at 7 days. If the isolate is suspected to be *Trichophyton verrucosum*, incubate the tubes at 37°C for the same period of time.

3)   The requirement for a growth substance is seen as weaker growth or an absence of growth in the absence of that substance. The growth in each tube is evaluated as follows:

   4+   good growth

   2+   intermediate growth

   ±   trace

   0   absence of growth

4)   It is possible, at the time of test evaluation, to suspect that chemical contamination of the *Trichophyton* agars during the process of inoculation has led to a false result. Inoculating a second series of media starting with inoculum obtained from agar #1 eliminates this contamination by diluting it to an insignificant level.

Quality control

Trichophyton tonsurans	growth stimulated by thiamine
Trichophyton verrucosum	growth dependent on thiamine and inositol

Bibliography
Georg, Camp, 1957

Table V. Growth of some dermatophytes on *Trichophyton* agars.

Species	Agar #						
	1	2	3	4	5	6	7
T. concentricum (50% of strains)	4+	4+	4+	4+			
T. concentricum (50% of strains)	2+	2+	4+	4+			
T. equinum var. *equinum*	0				4+		
T. equinum var. *autotrophicum*	4+				4+		
M. ferrugineum	4+	4+	4+	4+			
M. gallinae						4+	4+
T. megninii						1+	4+
T. mentagrophytes	4+	4+	4+	4+			
T. rubrum	4+	4+	4+	4+			
T. schoenleinii	4+	4+	4+	4+			
T. soudanense	±/1+	±/1+	±/1+	±/1+			
T. tonsurans	±/1+	±/1+	4+	4+			
T. verrucosum (84% of strains)	0	±	4+	0			
T. verrucosum (16% of strains)	0	0	4+	4+			
T. violaceum	±	±	4+	4+			

Composition

#1 : base (vitamin-free casein)
#2 : agar #1 + inositol
#3 : agar #1 + inositol + thiamine
#4 : agar #1 + thiamine
#5 : agar #1 + nicotinic acid (niacine)
#6 : base (ammonium nitrate)
#7 : agar #6 + histidine

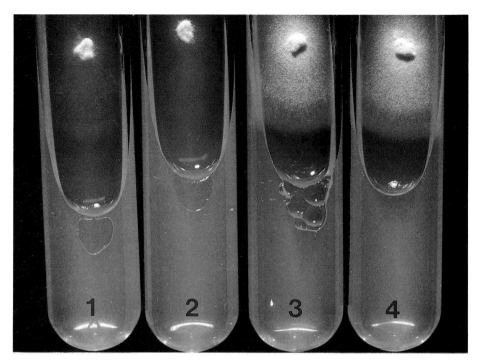

Figure 97.1 *Trichophyton tonsurans.* Growth stimulated by thiamine (partial dependence).

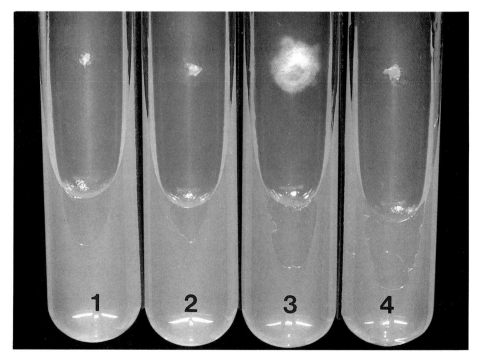

Figure 97.2 *Trichophyton verrucosum.* Growth absent or very weak in the absence of thiamine and inositol (total dependence).

248

Hydrolysis of urea

Objective
This is a test used primarily to distinguish *Trichophyton rubrum* and *T. menta-grophytes*. It may also be useful in the identification of some other dermato-phytes.

Principle
Urea hydrolysis in Christensen's medium causes a rise in pH following the for-mation of ammonia. This character is sometimes variable and cannot be used as a conclusive criterion in the identification of dermatophytes.

Method
1)   Inoculate a slant of Christensen's urea agar with a fragment of the colony.

2)   Incubate at 25°C for 7 days.

3)   A positive reaction is seen in a change of the original yellowish color of the medium to red.

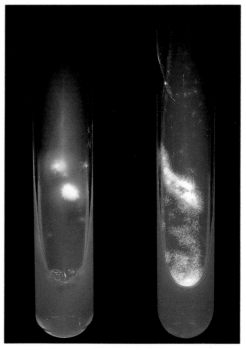

Figure 98.   Urease negative growth of *Trichophyton rubrum* (left) and urease posi-tive growth of *Trichophyton mentagrophytes* (right) on Christensen's urea agar.

249

Quality control

T. mentagrophytes	positive reaction (red)
T. rubrum	negative reaction (yellowish)

Bibliography
McGinnis, 1980
Weitzman, Kane, 1992

Hair perforation (in vitro)

Objective
Differentiates certain dermatophytes, particularly *Trichophyton rubrum* and *T. mentagrophytes*. It is most useful in the case of atypical isolates.

Principle
Some species of dermatophytes produce specialized hyphae called "perforating organs", capable of perforating hair *in vitro*.

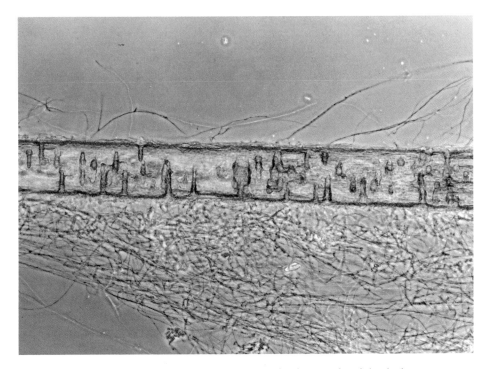

Figure 99. Cone shaped perforations to the long axis of the hair (*Trichophyton mentagrophytes*).

Method

1)   Pipette 25 ml of deionized water into a petri dish and add 2-3 drops of 10% yeast extract.

2)   Place on the water surface some fragments of sterilised hairs, originally from a prepubescent child, previously cut into 1 cm long segments and sterilised in an autoclave at 121°C for 15 minutes.

3)   Inoculate the hairs with small inoculum pieces from the dermatophyte colony under investigation.

4)   Incubate at 25°C for 28 days. Examine every 7 days.

5)   Mount some hair segments in a drop of water between a slide and a cover slip, and examine under the microscope at 100X.

6)   The test is positive when cone shaped perforations are observed perpendicular to the long axis of the hair. Most isolates of *T. mentagrophytes* are positive within 7 days.

Quality control

T. mentagrophytes	perforations present
T. rubrum	perforations absent

Bibliography
Rebell, Taplin, 1970

Reaction on bromcresol purple (BCP)-milk solids-glucose agar

Objective
Differentiates certain dermatophytes, particularly *Trichophyton rubrum, T. mentagrophytes*, and *Microsporum persicolor*.

Principle
Certain dermatophytes utilize the casein present in BCP-milk solids-glucose within 7 days in a way that results in the alkalinization of the medium (ammonification). In addition, some cause a broad zone of hydrolytic clearing (peptonization) to appear around the colonies.

Method

1)   Inoculate a BCP-milk solids-glucose slant with a small fragment from the colony under investigation.

2)   Incubate at 25°C for 7 days.

3)   Note any change in pH, the colony growth rate, and the formation of a zone of hydrolysis. Alkalinization of the medium is seen as a change of the original light blue color to dark blue or purple. Clearing hydrolysis results in a broad, clearly delineated, transparent zone around the edge of the colony in the otherwise opaque medium. If the pH indicator becomes yellow, this usually signals hidden contamination by bacteria or yeasts. The test isolate must then be decontaminated in order to obtain a valid result. Note that acidification may also be caused by filamentous fungi other than dermatophytes.

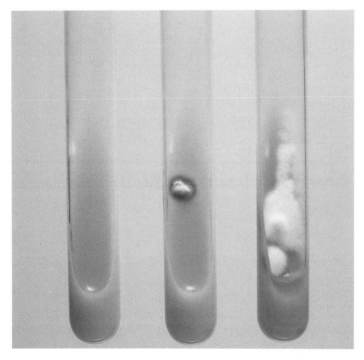

Figure 100.   BCP milk solids glucose agar. From left to right: uninoculated medium, *Trichophyton rubrum* and *Trichophyton mentagrophytes*.

Quality control

T. rubrum	no change of pH and restricted growth
T. mentagrophytes	alkalinization and profuse growth

Bibliography
Summerbell, Rosenthal, Kane, 1988
Weitzman, Kane, 1991

Stimulation of pigment production on potato glucose agar

Objective
Assists in the identification of certain dermatophytes (*Trichophyton rubrum, Microsporum audouinii, M. canis*) when they fail to produce characteristic pigment on Sabouraud glucose agar.

Principle
Potato glucose agar stimulates the production of characteristic pigments in the dermatophytes mentioned above.

Method
1)   Inoculate potato glucose agar with a fragment of the isolate under investigation.

2)   Incubate at 25°C for 14 days.

3)   Examine the cultures at 7 days and, if necessary, at 14 days. Note the color of the colony reverse.

Quality control

T. rubrum	red pigment on the colony reverse
T. mentagrophytes	yellow to brown pigment on the colony reverse
M. audouinii	salmon pigment on the colony reverse
M. canis	yellow orange pigment on the colony reverse

Bibliography
Rebell, Taplin, 1970

Probe technique for the identification of dimorphic fungi

Objective

To rapidly identify the dimorphic fungi *Histoplasma capsulatum*, *Blastomyces dermatitidis*, and *Coccidioides immitis*.

Principle

By means of a nucleic acid hybridization technique, the above fungi can be identified definitively within a few hours. The molecular probes sold commercially use a chemiluminescent detection principle (GenProbe, Inc., San Diego, California). They are both highly sensitive and highly specific.

Method

> Warning! Given the danger of infection by conidia of the fungi tested, it is recommended to carry out the initial stage of this procedure in a biological safety cabinet in a containment laboratory.

1) Grind a small fragment of the colony in 200 μl of lysis buffer. Close the tube tightly.

2) Sonicate the suspension in an ultrasound generator for 15 minutes in order to lyse the cells and liberate ribonucleic acid.

3) Heat to 95°C for 10 minutes to denature the RNA.

4) Proceed to the hybridization step by adding the probe to 100 μl of the lysate suspension; incubate at 60°C for 15 minutes.

5) Neutralize the unhybridized probe by adding 300 μl of neutralization buffer.

6) Measure the amount of hybridized probe with the aid of a luminometer.

Quality control

The use of strains of dimorphic fungi is recommended for both positive and negative controls.

Bibliography

Hall, Pratt-Rippin, Washington, 1992
Padhye, Smith, McLaughlin, Standard, Kaufman, 1992
Stockman, Clark, Hunt, Roberts, 1993

Immuno-identification (exoantigen) technique for dimorphic fungi

Objective
To identify rapidly the dimorphic fungi *Histoplasma capsulatum*, *Blastomyces dermatitidis*, and *Coccidioides immitis* by detecting specific exoantigens.

Principle
The dimorphic fungi contain extractable, soluble exoantigens which react in immunodiffusion trials with specific antibodies formed in the serum of infected animals or in monoclonal antibody production systems. With the aid of commercially available kits (Immuno-Mycologics, Norman, OK; Meridian Diagnostics, Cincinnati, OH) it is possible to study the reactions of antigens extracted from test isolates and to confirm or exclude the identification of the three dimorphic fungi mentioned above. This technique is reputed to be virtually 100% specific.

Method

> **Warning!** Given the danger of infection by conidia of the fungi tested, it is recommended to carry out the first three steps of this procedure in a biological safety cabinet in a containment laboratory.

1) Extract the exoantigens of the test isolate by completely covering a colony on a Sabouraud glucose slant with 6 to 10 ml of a 0.02% merthiolate solution. The colony must exceed 1.5 cm in diameter.

2) Leave to steep for 18-24 hours at room temperature.

3) Collect the supernatant and, for greater security, filter through a 0.45 μm membrane filter to assure sterility.

4) Concentrate the antigen solution with the aid of a Minicon Macrosolute B-15 concentrator (Amicon, Inc., Beverly, MN).

5) Place the concentrated exoantigens and the kit's control antigens in the peripheral wells of an immunodiffusion grid and confront them with the kit's specific antiserum placed in the center well. (Follow manufacturer's instructions; the kit may require the antiserum to be added prior to the addition of the antigens).

6) Incubate in a humid chamber at 25°C for 18-24 hours.

7) Look for the presence of a continuous band of identity between the precipitate bands from the test isolate and those from the reference antigen. The presence of the HS, F or HL antigens confirms the identification of *C. immitis*. The H and/or the M antigen confirms *H. capsulatum*, and the A antigen confirms *B. dermatitidis* (southern African isolates excepted).

Note: Occasionally, the quantity of exoantigens obtained from the colony on the slant is insufficient. If the results of the test are suspected to be falsely negative because of this factor, the test must be repeated using a larger colony or using material obtained after growing the test isolate in brain-heart infusion broth under agitation.

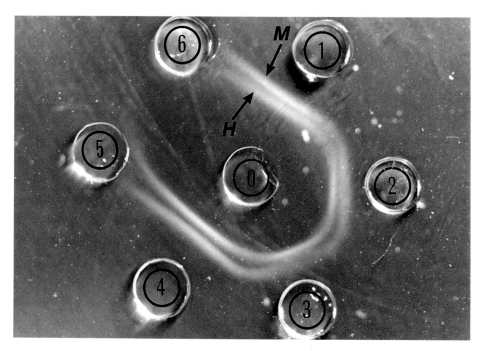

Figure 101.   Identification of *Histoplasma capsulatum*; presence of H and M bands of identity. 0, control antiserum; 1 and 4, control antigens; 2 and 3, culture extract from *H. capsulatum*; 5 and 6, culture extract from a negative culture.

Quality control
Each test done necessitates the utilization of the control antigens furnished in the kit. Exoantigens extracted from known isolates of dimorphic fungi should be used occasionally to verify the extraction technique.

Bibliography
Kaufman, Reiss, 1986
Standard, Kaufman, Whaley, 1985

Conversion of dimorphic fungi from the filamentous phase to the yeast phase

Objective
To confirm the identification of the dimorphic fungi *Blastomyces dermatitidis*, *Histoplasma capsulatum*, *Paracoccidioides brasiliensis*, and *Sporothrix schenckii*.

Principle
Dimorphic fungi are usually isolated in their filamentous phase at temperatures between 25°C and 30°C. To confirm their identification it is often necessary to verify that they convert to a yeast phase at 37°C on rich media. It is also possible to obtain spherules of *Coccidioides immitis* in vitro at 40°C but this technique is of little use in the diagnostic laboratory. Exoantigen or probe studies are the best ways of confirming the identification of this organism.

Method

> **Warning!** Given the danger of infection by conidia of the fungi tested, it is recommended to carry out these procedures in a biological safety cabinet in a containment laboratory, except in the case of *S. schenckii*.

There exist a variety of specialized media for obtaining the yeast forms of dimorphic fungi. Although brain-heart infusion agar with 10% sheep blood is generally adequate to effect the conversions, certain specialized media like Blasto "D" medium for *B. dermatitidis*, as well as blood-glucose-cysteine medium and Kurung-Yegian medium for *H. capsulatum*, are reputed to be of greater efficacy.

1) Inoculate the slant of conversion medium with a fragment of the colony to be tested. If the slant appears somewhat dry, moisten it with a few drops of sterile brain-heart broth or sterile water.

2) Incubate at 37°C in aerobic atmosphere or in 5% CO_2.

3) After 3-7 days of incubation, transfer a small sample from the new colony to a drop of lactophenol-cotton blue on a slide and examine under the microscope for the presence of some yeast cells. If yeasts are absent, inoculate a second slant with inoculum obtained from the periphery of the colony growing on the first slant of conversion medium. It is sometimes necessary to repeat this operation three or four times to obtain the formation of yeasts.

4) *B. dermatitidis* produces large yeasts, 10-15 μm in diameter, with refractile walls, and with buds characteristically forming on a broad base. This usually occurs in a week or less, often within 72 hours. *H. capsulatum* produces small budding yeasts, 2- 4 μm in diameter, budding on a narrow base. Their formation may require several weeks of incubation. *P. brasiliensis* produces yeasts with multipolar, satellite budding. *S. schenckii* produces yeast with cigar-shaped buds, often within a few days of incubation.

Quality control

Given the danger of infection associated with manipulating these microorganisms, routine performance of control studies with sporulated cultures is not recommended.

Bibliography
McGinnis, 1980
Moser, Lyon, Greer, 1988

Assimilation of potassium nitrate

Objective
To differentiate *Wangiella dermatitidis* from *Exophiala jeanselmei*

Principle
The assimilation of potassium nitrate as a sole source of nitrogen brings about the alkalinization of the culture medium.

Method
1) Inoculate the potassium nitrate medium by streaking a slant or by placing a fragment of the test colony onto the surface.

2) Incubate at 25-30°C for a period of 7 days.

3) A positive reaction is signalled by a change of the medium color from yellow to deep blue.

Quality control

E. jeanselmei	positive assimilation (deep blue)
W. dermatitidis	negative assimilation (yellow)

Bibliography
Steadham, Geis, Simmank, 1986
Dixon, Polak-Wyss, 1991

Thermotolerance

Objective

Aids in the identification of numerous species of fungi. As a general rule, the absence of growth of a fungus at 37°C indicates that it is unlikely to be the cause of a deep infection of humans.

Principle

The maximum temperature of growth is a stable characteristic in numerous species of filamentous fungi.

Table VI. Thermotolerance of certain medically important fungi.

Species	Temperature (°C)				
	30°	37°	40°	45°	54°
Absidia corymbifera	+	+	+	+	−
Aspergillus fumigatus	+	+	+	+	−
Bipolaris spicifera	+	+	+	−	−
Cladosporium carrionii	+	±	−	−	−
Dactylaria gallopava	+	+	+.	−	
Exserohilum mcginnisii	+	+	+	−	−
Exophiala jeanselmei	+	+	−	−	−
Fonsecaea pedrosoi	+	+	−	−	−
Microsporum persicolor	+	+w	−	−	−
Rhizomucor pusillus	+	+	+	+	+
Rhizopus arrhizus	+	+	+	±	−
Rhizopus rhizopodiformis	+	+	+	+	−
Scedosporium apiospermum	+	+	+	−	−
Scedosporium prolificans	+	+	+	+	−
Scolecobasidium constrictum	+	−	−	−	−
Trichophyton terrestre	+	−	−	−	−
Trichophyton verrucosum	+	+*	−	−	−
Wangiella dermatitidis	+	+	+	−	−
Xylohypha bantiana	+	+	+	−	−

w, weak; * *better growth at 37°C than at 25°C.*

Method

1) Inoculate a minimum of two Sabouraud glucose agar slants with a fragment of the test colony; the size of the inoculum pieces should be similar in both tubes.

2) Incubate one of the tubes at 25°C as a control ensuring viable inoculum, and the remaining tube(s) at 37, 40, 45, or 54°C according to the organism queried.

3) The duration of the incubation may vary from 2 to 7 days, depending on the growth rate of the fungus.

4) Assure that the organism has grown at 25°C; then determine the higher temperatures at which the fungus has grown. In some cases, it is useful to note the size of the colonies.

Quality control

Aspergillus fumigatus	good growth at 48°C
Rhizomucor pusillus	growth at 54°C
Trichophyton terrestre	no growth at 37°C
Trichophyton verrucosum	growth more rapid at 37°C than at 25°C
Wangiella dermatitidis	growth at 40°C

Bibliography

Dixon, Polak-Wyss, 1991
McGinnis, 1980
Rebell, Taplin, 1970

Preparation of specimens for microscopic examination

Objective

To effect the identification of filamentous fungi by examining their microscopic structures.

Principle

The most simple technique consists in placing a fragment of the colony between slide and cover slip. This approach is rapid and often adequate for identification. Delicate fungal structures, however, are often broken by this process, rendering identification difficult.

The adhesive tape technique assists in maintaining the integrity of fungal structures by fixing them on the adhesive surface of a piece of transparent (NOT frosted) tape.

The slide culture technique consists in growing a microcolony of the fungus on a slide or on a cover slip. The developing fungal colony adheres to the surface of the glass and facilitates the observation of intact conidial structures.

Methods

A)   Direct examination of a portion of the colony

1)   With the aid of a sterile needle, detach a small fragment of the colony to be identified and place it in a drop of lactophenol-cotton blue.

2)   Using two needles, gently spread apart the material to be examined.

3)   Cover the preparation with a cover slip and press gently to flatten the preparation.

4)   Examine microscopically.

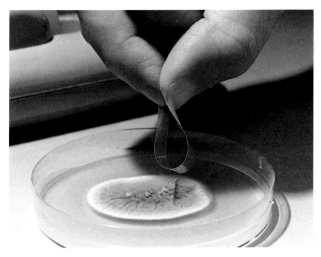

Figure 102.1 Adhesive tape technique.

B)   Adhesive tape technique

1)   Cut a piece of adhesive cellulose tape and fold it back on itself with the adhesive side turned outward. To hold on to the ends of the loop, forceps may be useful.

2)   Press the adhesive side of the tape onto the surface of the colony and pull it away. The aerial hyphae of the colony will remain glued onto the tape surface.

3)   Place the tape in a drop of lactophenol-cotton blue previously placed at the center of a glass slide.

4)   Examine microscopically.

C)   Slide culture technique (Riddell method)

1)   Place a bent, U-shaped glass rod in the bottom of a sterile petri plate. Place a clean, sterile slide on the glass rod and then place a block of medium at the center of this slide.

2)   Inoculate the sides of the medium block with small pieces of the culture to be identified.

3)   Place a cover slip sterilized by rapid passage over a flame onto the block of medium.

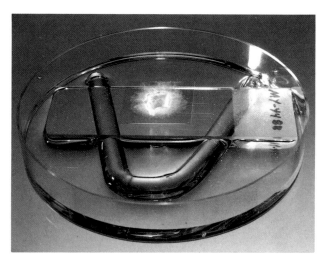

Figure 102.2 Classic Riddell slide culture technique.

4)   Pipette around 5 ml of sterile water onto the bottom of the petri plate to ensure maintenance of humidity, and then close the petri plate.

5)   Incubate at an optimal temperature, generally 25°C.

6)   The slide may be taken out of the petri plate and examined under the microscope at regular intervals to determine whether sporulation has occurred.

7)   When the culture has sporulated, lift the cover slip from the medium block and fix it by passing it rapidly in close proximity to a burner flame. Mount it by placing it over a drop of cotton blue or other mounting fluid on a glass slide.

8)   It is also possible to mount the portion of the culture which remains attached to the slide after disposing of the block of medium.

9)   These preparations may be sealed by applying a layer of nail polish around the perimeter of the cover slip. Such preparations, if well sealed, may remain in good condition for 1- 5 years.

D   Simplified slide culture technique (Harris method, modified)

1)   Beginning with a petri plate of growth medium, cut two small blocks of medium from one side of the plate and place them on the surface of the medium near the opposite side.

264

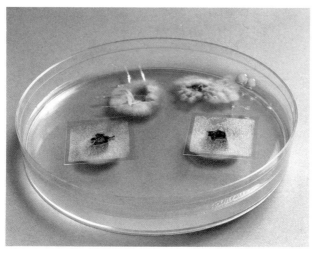

Figure 102.3   Simplified slide culture technique.

2)   Inoculate the sides of the two blocks with small pieces of the culture to be studied.

3)   Place a cover slip sterilized by rapid passage through a flame onto each of the two blocks, close the petri plate, and incubate.

4)   When appropriate, fix and mount the cover slips as described above.

Remarks

1)   When cover slips are being mounted, do not use more than a small quantity of mounting fluid between slide and cover slip. When the thickness of the preparation is minimized, most of the fungal structures will be in the same plane, making examination easier. This detail is especially important for photography. In addition, an excess of liquid will prevent proper sealing of the cover slip in any attempt to make a permanent mount of the preparation.

2)   More enduring mounts can be produced by placing a small drop of lactophenol cotton blue on the coverslip bearing the fungal growth and covering it with a second cover slip of smaller size. This whole preparation is then placed with the smaller coverslip facing downward onto a drop of balsam or other permanent mounting material in the center of a slide.

Bibliography

Koneman, Roberts, 1985

Purification of isolates contaminated by bacteria

Objective
To purify bacterially contaminated cultures prior to proceeding to analyses requiring a pure culture.

Principle
The elimination of bacteria is brought about by culture on media amended with antibacterials or by culture in acid media.

Methods

A)   Antibacterials

1)   Inoculate a selective medium containing several antibacterials: chloramphenicol (50 mg/l), penicillin (20,000- 50,000 units/l) gentamicin (5 mg/l) and/or streptomycin (40 mg/l).

2)   Incubate at 25°C for several days.

3)   Verify the efficacy of the inhibitory agent by examining the new fungal colonies by means of a gram stain preparation.

4)   In the event of a failure, repeat using other antibiotics or proceed to decontaminate in acid medium.

B)   Hydrochloric acid

1)   Prepare a suspension of the culture to be decontaminated in 1 or 2 ml of sterile deionized water.

2)   To each of four tubes containing 5 ml of Sabouraud glucose broth, add respectively 1, 2, 3 and 4 drops of 1N hydrochloric acid.

3)   Inoculate each tube with 1 drop of the contaminated culture.

4)   Incubate at 25°C as long as is necessary to obtain visible growth in the first tube (control).

5)   From each of the tubes, take about 0.1 ml of broth and streak it onto a Sabouraud glucose plate or slant.

6)   Incubate at 25°C and examine for the presence of pure, well isolated colonies.

Quality control
The effectiveness of the antibiotics incorporated in media can be verified with the aid of known susceptible bacterial strains.

Bibliography
McGinnis, 1980

Conservation of isolates

Objective
To assure the viability and phenotypic stability of isolates put in culture collections. These isolates may then be used in later studies, as quality control isolates, or as reference vouchers.

Principle
The principal methods of conservation are lyophilization and freezing. A more simple technique involves conserving the isolate in suspension in sterile deionized water. In any case, the object of the technique is to stop or greatly retard the metabolism of the cells during the period in which cultures are stored, and at the same time to preserve their viability and their characteristics.

Methods
Conidia and spores are among the most resistant fungal structures, and, for this reasons, give the best results with each of the techniques described below. Sporulating cultures are prepared on potato glucose agar or any other medium favouring sporulation. Nonsporulating strains cannot be lyophilized, since the hyphae are usually too fragile to withstand this procedure. Such isolates are better conserved in sterile water or in the freezer. It is necessary to use young, actively growing cells in the preparation of suspensions for long term storage.

A)   Conservation in sterile deionized water

1)   Prepare a dense suspension of conidia, spores or hyphae in 1 ml of sterile deionized water, while carefully avoiding the transfer of growth medium along with the fungal material.

2)   Retain this suspension at room temperature, in a small, hermetically closed vial.

267

3)   This technique allows most isolates of medical mycological interest to be conserved for a period of between 1 and 5 years.

4)   To obtain a fresh subculture of the organism, shake the tube and transfer 1 drop of the suspension onto Sabouraud glucose agar.

B)   Freezing

1)   Prepare a dense suspension of conidia, spores or hyphae in a cryotube containing 0.5 to 1 ml of 10% glycerol and a dozen porous, sterile glass beads.

2)   Shake the contents of the tube well for 30 seconds and remove the bulk of the liquid from the cryotube with the aid of a Pasteur pipette.

3)   Freeze the glass beads by placing them immediately in a -60°C freezer. A rapid freezing process minimizes the damage to cells during this critical step.

4)   The frozen cells remain viable for 10 years or more.

5)   When reviving the frozen material, it is necessary to ensure that the thawing of the cells occurs as rapidly as possible. To obtain a fresh culture, remove a glass bead from the cryotube and place it on medium already at room temperature. Return the cryotube to the freezer immediately to avoid warming of the remaining beads.

C)   Lyophilization

1)   Prepare a thick suspension of conidia or spores in autoclaved skim milk and transfer into a lyophilization ampule.

2)   Lyophilize the suspension.

3)   Store the ampules, if possible, at 2-8°C.

4)   Lyophilized strains may be conserved for a period of 10 years or more.

5) To rehydrate an isolate, suspend the contents of an ampule in 0.5 ml sterile deionized water and let the mixture stand for 30 minutes. Inoculate a tube of Sabouraud glucose broth with 0.4 ml of the preparation and a plate of Sabouraud glucose agar with the remaining drops of material.

Bibliography

Simione, Brown, 1991
Smith, 1991

Culture media and stains

In medical mycology, a variety of culture media are used for the isolation, identification and conservation of fungi. It is important to be familiar with the composition and characteristics of these media, because the selection of appropriate media for a given task is critical in diagnostic work.

Ingredients and preparation

Culture media of good quality are indispensable for assurance of adequate service in the diagnostic laboratory. To this end, when using commercial media, it is important to deal with reputable manufacturers with an efficient distribution network. Laboratories wishing to prepare their own media from commercial powdered formulations must do so in accordance with the manufacturer's instructions. The quality of water used, the thoroughness with which ingredients are dissolved or suspended and the temperature and duration of autoclaving are also factors which can affect the quality of the final product.

Quality control

Each new lot of culture medium, whether it has been purchased in a ready-to-use form or prepared by the user, must be quality controlled for its appearance, sterility, pH and performance. The performance of selective media can be evaluated by inoculating organisms susceptible and resistant to the inhibitory agents in the media. Differential media are evaluated with organisms known to produce positive and negative reactions. Media for isolation or for general use are evaluated for their ability to support optimal growth of selected isolates.

Storage

In general, culture media can be stored in the refrigerator at 2- 8 °C. It is better to invert petri plates and to enclose them in tightly closed plastic bags to prevent dehydration. Media in petri plates stored in this way usually remain in good condition for about 3 months, while semisolid or liquid media in well sealed screw-capped tubes may be kept for about 6 months. Certain media containing unstable substances (antibiotics, blood, vitamins or others) must be used more promptly.

Bibliography
Atlas, 1993
Miller, 1991
NCCLS, 1990

Blasto "D" medium

Composition

Glucose	7 g
Tween 80	0.2 ml
Potassium sulfate (K_2SO_4)	0.5 g
Magnesium citrate ($C_{12}H_{10}Mg_3O_{14}$)	1.5 g
Dipotassium phosphate (K_2HPO_4)	5 g
Asparagine	5.0 g
Casamino acids	3.0 g
Sodium chloride (NaCl)	0.85 g
Agar	15 g
Deionized water	1000 ml

Preparation

a) Mix the ingredients and adjust to pH 6.6. Bring to a boil to dissolve completely.
b) Pour into tubes.
c) Sterilize at 121°C for 15 minutes.
d) Cool in an inclined position.

Quality control

a) Appearance: medium colorless, transparent
b) final pH at 25°C: 6.6 ± 0.2
c) Performance:
  Blastomyces dermatitidis: yeast form at 37°C

Usage

A specialized medium for converting *B. dermatitidis* from its filamentous form to the yeast form.

Bibliography

Kane, 1984

Blood-glucose-cysteine agar

Composition

Tryptose blood agar base *	33 g
L-cysteine (hydrochlorate)	1 g
Defibrinated sheep blood	50 ml
Penicillin (100,000 U/ml)	10 ml
Deionized water	990 ml

Preparation

a) Mix the ingredients (excepting the blood and penicillin) and bring to a boil to dissolve completely.

272

b) Sterilize at 121°C for 15 minutes.
c) Cool to 50°C and add the blood and penicillin.

Quality control
a) Appearance: bright red medium, opaque
b) Final pH at 25°C: 7.2 ± 0.2
c) Performance:
    Histoplasma capsulatum   yeast form at 37°C

Usage
Medium used to promote the conversion of the filamentous phase of *H. capsulatum*, *Blastomyces dermatitidis*, *Paracoccidioides brasiliensis* a n d *Sporothrix schenckii* to the yeast phase.

Bibliography
Kwon-Chung, Bennett, 1992

    * *medium available commercially*

Brain-heart infusion agar*

Composition

Calf brain infusion	200 g
Beef heart infusion	250 g
Peptone	10 g
Glucose	2 g
Sodium chloride (NaCl)	5 g
Disodium phosphate (Na$_2$HPO$_4$)	2.5 g
Agar	15 g
Deionized water	1000 ml

Preparation
a) Mix the ingredients and bring to a boil to dissolve completely.
b) Sterilize at 121°C for 15 minutes.

Modifications
a) enriched with 5-10% defibrinated sheep blood
b) with chloramphenicol (50 mg/l)

Quality control
a) Appearance: solid medium, amber, transparent
                             or (if blood added) bright red, opaque
b) Final pH at 25°C: 7.4 ± 0.2

c) Performance:

Candida albicans	growth
Sporothrix schenckii	conversion to yeast phase at 37°C
Staphylococcus epidermidis	partial or total inhibition on medium with chloramphenicol

Usage

A rich medium used with or without antibiotics for the isolation of pathogenic fungi from clinical specimens. The enriched version with sheep blood also serves in the conversion of dimorphic fungi to the yeast phase.

    * *Medium available commercially.*

Bromcresol purple-milk solids-glucose agar
(BCP-casein-dextrose agar)

Composition—Solution A:

Powdered skim milk	80 g
Bromcresol purple 1.6% (diluted in ethanol)	2 ml
Deionized water	1000 ml

Composition—Solution B:

Glucose	40 g
Deionized water	200 ml

Composition—Solution C:

Agar	30 g
Deionized water	800 ml

Preparation

a) Make up solutions A and B and autoclave them separately at 115°C for 8 minutes.
b) Bring solution C to a boil to dissolve agar completely and autoclave at 121°C for 15 minutes.
c) Add solutions A and B into C, mix, cool to 50°C and adjust the pH to 6.6 with drops from a solution of 1N hydrochloric acid.
d) Pour aseptically into tubes and leave to cool in slanted position.

Quality control

a) Appearance: solid medium, slanted, sky blue, opaque

b) Final pH at 25°C: 6.6 ±0.1

c) Performance:

Trichophyton rubrum:	no change in pH and restricted growth in 7 days at 25°C.
Trichophyton mentagrophytes:	alkalinization and profuse growth in 7 days at 25°C

274

Usage

Differential medium used for identification of dermatophytes, especially to differentiate *T. rubrum* and *M. persicolor* from *T. mentagrophytes*.

Bibliography

Weitzman, Kane, 1991

Christensen urea agar*

Composition—Solution A:

Peptone	1 g
Glucose	1 g
Monopotassium phosphate (KH_2PO4)	2 g
Sodium chloride (NaCl)	5 g
Urea	20 g
Phenol red	0.012 g
Deionized water	100 ml

Composition—Solution B:

Agar	5 g
Deionized water	900 ml

Preparation

a) Make up solution A and, after solids are dissolved completely, sterilize by filtration.
b) Bring solution B to a boil to dissolve ingredients completely.
c) Sterilize solution B at 121°C for 15 minutes.
d) Cool the medium to 50°C and add solution A.
e) Dispense in tubes and cool in slanted position.

Quality control

a) Appearance: medium slanted, orange, transparent
b) Final pH at 25°C: 6.8 ± 0.2
c) Performance:
   Trichophyton mentagrophytes urease positive (red)
   Trichophyton rubrum urease negative (orange)

Usage

Medium useful for identifying certain dermatophytes, in particular *T. rubrum* and *T. mentagrophytes*.

Bibliography

McGinnis, 1980

* Medium available commercially

275

Cornmeal glucose agar

Composition

Cornmeal (infusion of)	40 g
Glucose	20 g
Purified agar	15 g
Deionized water	1000 ml

Preparation

a) Mix cornflour in the water. Heat 1 hour at 52°C or autoclave at 121°C for 10 minutes. Filter through cheesecloth and then through Whatman #2 filter paper.
b) Add the agar and bring to a boil to dissolve. Add the glucose, mix and bring the volume up to 1000 ml with deionized water.
c) Sterilize at 121°C for 15 minutes.

Quality control

a) Appearance: whitish solid medium, translucent
b) Final pH at 25°C: 6.0 ± 0.2
c) Performance:

Trichophyton rubrum	red pigment on the colony reverse
Trichophyton mentagrophytes	brown pigment on the colony reverse

Usage

A medium which stimulates production of red pigment in strains of *T. rubrum* failing to produce this pigment on Sabouraud glucose agar.

Bibliography

Bocobo, 1949

Czapek-Dox agar*

Composition

Sodium nitrate (NaNO$_3$)	3 g
Dipotassium phosphate (K$_2$HPO$_4$)	1 g
Magnesium sulfate (MgSO$_4$.7H$_2$0)	0.5 g
Potassium chloride (KCl)	0.5 g
Ferrous sulfate (FeSO$_4$.7H$_2$0)	0.01 g
Sucrose	30 g
Agar	15 g
Deionized water	1000 ml

Preparation

a) Mix the ingredients and bring to a boil to dissolve completely.
b) Sterilize at 121°C for 15 minutes.
c) Pour into petri plates.

Quality control

a) Appearance: pale amber, solid transparent medium, sometimes with crystals

b) Final pH at 25°C: 7.3 ± 0.2.

c) Performance:
   Aspergillus flavus growth, yellow green colony

Usage

A reference medium for the identification of *Aspergillus* species.

   * *Medium available commercially*

Kurung-Yegian medium

Composition—Solution A:

Potato flour	5 g
Deionized water	500 ml

Composition—Solution B:

Whole egg	250 ml
Egg yolk (50% enrichment)	500 ml

Preparation

a) Mix solution A without heating, adjust pH to 5.0 and then heat until dissolved.

b) Sterilize at 121°C for 15 minutes.

c) Cool to 50°C in a water bath.

d) Let the whole, unbroken eggs stand in 70% ethanol for 15-30 minutes.

e) Prepare solution B by breaking open the eggs and mixing them aseptically in a blender with the egg yolk enrichment.

f) Add solution A to solution B and mix.

g) Apportion into tubes and slant.

h) Allow to set 25 minutes at 82°C in the autoclave (isothermal cycle).

Quality control

a) Appearance: solid slant, yellow, opaque

b) Final pH at 25°C: 6.6 ± 0.2

c) Performance:
   Histoplasma capsulatum yeast form at 37°C

Usage

An egg medium favoring the conversion of *H. capsulatum* to the yeast phase. Often useful also for converting *Blastomyces dermatitidis*.

Bibliography
Kurung, Yegian, 1954
Segretain, Drouhet, Mariat, 1984

Lactritmel agar (Borelli's Medium)

Composition

Whole wheat flour	14 g
Powdered skim milk	14 g
Honey	7 g
Agar	14 g
Deionized water	1000 ml

Preparation

a) Mix the ingredients and bring to a boil.
b) Sterilize at 121°C for 15 minutes.
c) Pour in petri plates.

Quality control

a) Appearance: solid medium, whitish, opaque, with brown particles
b) Final pH at 25°C: 6.8 ± 0.2
c) Performance:
   Microsporum canis   abundant sporulation

Usage

A medium favoring the sporulation of dermatophytes, particularly *M. canis*. Also used for morphological examination of dematiaceous fungi.

Bibliography
Salkin, 1989
Segretain, Drouhet, Mariat, 1984

Mycosel/Mycobiotic agar*

Composition

Peptone	10 g
Glucose	10 g
Agar	15 g
Cycloheximide	0.4 g
Chloramphenicol	0.05 g
Deionized water	1000 ml

Preparation

a) Mix the ingredients and bring to a boil to dissolve completely.
b) Sterilize at 121°C for 15 minutes.

Quality control

a) Appearance: a yellowish, transparent, solid medium
b) Final pH at 25°C: 6.9 ± 0.2
c) Performance:

Trichophyton verrucosum	growth
Aspergillus flavus	partial or complete inhibition
Staphylococcus epidermidis	partial or complete inhibition

Usage

A selective medium principally used for the primary isolation of dermatophytes. For the isolation of other fungi, it is necessary to use this medium in combination with other media not containing cycloheximide, as this antibiotic inhibits the growth of numerous potentially pathogenic yeasts and filamentous fungi.

> * *Medium available commercially (Mycosel [BBL, Becton Dickinson, Cockeysville, MD] and Mycobiotic [Difco Laboratories, Detroit, MI] are registered trade names; similar media are sold under other names by numerous manufacturers). The concentration of cycloheximide and the pH may vary slightly according to the manufacturer.*

Nitrate agar

Composition

Potassium nitrate (KNO_3)	1.4 g
Yeast carbon base *	1.6 g
Bromthymol blue	0.12 g
Purified agar	16 g
Deionized water	1000 ml

Preparation

a) Mix the ingredients and bring to a boil to dissolve completely.
b) Adjust the pH to 5.9-6.0.

c) Pour into tubes.
d) Sterilize at 121°C for 15 minutes.
e) Cool in an inclined position.

Quality control

a) Appearance: solid medium, slanted, yellow, transparent
b) Final pH at 25°C: 5.9-6.0
c) Performance:
   Exophiala jeanselmei positive assimilation (dark blue)
   Wangiella dermatitidis negative assimilation (yellow)

Usage

A medium used in the differentiation of the dematiaceous fungi E. *jeanselmei* and W. *dermatitidis*.

Bibliography

Salkin, 1989

* *Medium available commercially.*

Potato flake agar

Composition

Potato flakes	20 g
Glucose	10 g
Agar	15 g
Deionized water	1000 ml

Preparation

a) Mix the ingredients and bring to a boil.
b) Sterilize at 121°C for 15 minutes.

Quality control

a) Appearance: colorless, translucent solid medium
b) Performance: no evaluation is necessary before usage

Usage

Favors the sporulation of fungi.

Bibliography

Atlas, 1993

Potato glucose agar *
(Potato dextrose agar)

Composition

Potatoes	200 g
Glucose	10 g
Agar	18 g
Deionized water	1000 ml

Preparation

a) Peel the potatoes, cut into cubes and boil in water for one hour.
b) Filter through cheesecloth, add glucose and agar; bring to a boil to dissolve agar completely and filter again on Whatman #2 filter paper.
c) Adjust the volume to 1 litre.
d) Sterilize at 121°C for 15 minutes.

Quality control

a) Appearance: colorless or lightly yellow, solid medium, transparent or translucent
b) Final pH at 25°C: 5.6 ± 0.2
c) Performance:

Microsporum audouinii	salmon pigment in colony reverse
Trichophyton rubrum	deep red pigment in colony reverse
Trichophyton mentagrophytes	brown pigment in colony reverse

Usage

A medium favoring sporulation of most fungi of medical interest. Stimulates production of red pigment in *T. rubrum*, salmon pink pigment in *M. audouinii* and yellow pigment in *M. canis*.

* Medium available commercially

Rice medium

Composition

White rice, unenriched	8 g
Deionized water	25 ml

Preparation

a) Mix the ingredients in an erlenmeyer.
b) Sterilize at 121°C for 15 minutes.

Quality control

a) Appearance: cooked rice grains

b) Performance:

    Microsporum canis   good growth, yellow pigment, abundant sporulation

    Microsporum audouinii   no or weak growth, brownish discoloration

Usage

A medium used for the identification of *M. audouinii* and sometimes also for nonsporulating isolates of *M. canis*.

Bibliography

Rebell, Taplin, 1970

Vanbreuseghem, 1978

*Sabouraud glucose agar**

Composition

Peptone	10 g
Glucose	40 g
Agar	15 g
Deionized water	1000 ml

Preparation

a) Mix the ingredients and bring to a boil to dissolve completely.

b) Sterilize at 121°C for 15 minutes.

c) Dispense into tubes or petri plates.

Modification

With chloramphenicol (50 mg/l)

Quality control

a) Appearance: solid medium, amber, transparent

b) Final pH at 25°C: 5.6 ± 0.2

c) Performance:

    Trichophyton mentagrophytes   growth

    Staphylococcus epidermidis   partial or complete inhibition on medium with chloramphenicol

Usage

A medium recommended for the examination of colony morphology of dermatophytes. When it is used for the isolation of pathogenic fungi from clinical specimens which are not normally sterile, it is preferably supplemented with chloramphenicol, even though its somewhat acidic pH tends to deter bacterial contaminants.

* Medium available commercially

Sabouraud glucose agar, modified *
(Emmons' modification)

Composition

Peptone	10 g
Glucose	20 g
Agar	15 g
Deionized water	1000 ml

Preparation

a) Mix the ingredients and bring to a boil to dissolve completely.
b) Sterilize at 121°C for 15 minutes.

Modification

With chloramphenicol (50 mg/l).

Quality control

a) Appearance: amber, solid medium, transparent
b) Final pH at 25°C: 7.0 ± 0.2
c) Performance:
  Trichophyton mentagrophytes growth
  Staphylococcus epidermidis partial or complete inhibition on medium with chloramphenicol

Usage

Sabouraud's medium modified by Emmons to adjust the pH to 7.0 and the concentration of glucose to 2%. The changes were to optimize the utility of the medium in primary isolation and in stimulating sporulation of isolates.

* Medium available commercially

Sabouraud glucose broth*

Composition

Peptone	10 g
Glucose	20 g
Deionized water	1000 ml

Preparation

a) Mix the ingredients and dissolve completely.
b) Sterilize at 121°C for 15 minutes.

Quality control

a) Appearance: amber broth, transparent
b) Final pH at 25°C: 5.6 ± 0.2
c) Performance:
   Trichophyton mentagrophytes   growth

Usage

Used with added hydrochloric acid in the technique for purification of bacterially contaminated isolates (q.v.). It may also serve to revive certain aging fungal cultures, for which a large piece of the previous colony is placed into the broth, or the broth is added directly to the surface of the culture to be regenerated. Incubate 3-4 weeks.

Bibliography

McGinnis, 1980

   * *medium available commercially*

Soil extract agar

Composition

Garden soil	500 g
Glucose	2 g
Yeast extract	1 g
Monopotassium phosphate (KH_2PO_4)	0.5 g
Agar	15 g
Tap water	1000 ml

Preparation

a) Add garden soil to the water and autoclave for 3 hours at 121°C.
b) Allow to settle and filter through Whatman #2 filter paper.
c) Adjust the volume to 1 liter with tap water.
d) Mix the other ingredients into the soil infusion.
e) Adjust the pH to 7.0.
f) Bring to a boil to dissolve the agar.
g) Sterilize at 121°C for 15 minutes.

Quality control

a) Appearance: solid medium, brownish, transparent
b) Final pH at 25°C: 7.0 ± 0.2
c) Performance:
    Chrysosporium sp.   growth, abundant sporulation

Usage
Stimulates sporulation in some saprobic fungi.

Bibliography
McGinnis, 1980
Vanbreuseghem, 1978

*Trichophyton agars 1 to 7 ***

Composition

Trichophyton agar #1:

Casamino acids, vitamin-free	2.5 g
Glucose	40 g
Monopotassium phosphate (KH_2PO_4)	1.8 g
Magnesium sulfate ($MgSO_4.7H_2O$)	0.1 g
Agar	15 g
Deionized water	1000 ml

Medium #2: Medium #1 + inositol 50 mg
Medium #3: Medium #1 + inositol 50 mg + thiamine.HCl 0.2 mg
Medium #4: Medium #1 + thiamine.HCl 0.2 mg
Medium #5: Medium #1 + nicotinic acid (niacin) 2.0 mg

Trichophyton agar #6:

Ammonium nitrate (NH_4NO_3)	1.5 g
Glucose	40 g
Monopotassium phosphate (KH_2PO_4)	1.8 g
Magnesium sulfate ($MgSO_4.7H_2O$)	0.1 g
Agar	15 g
Deionized water	1000 ml

Medium #7: Medium #6 + histidine.HCl 30 mg

Preparation
a) Mix the ingredients and bring to a boil to dissolve completely.
b) Dispense in tubes.
c) Autoclave at 121°C for 15 minutes.
d) Cool in slanted position.

Quality control

a) Appearance: medium slanted, amber, transparent
b) Final pH at 25°C: 6.8 ± 0.2
c) Performance:

Media

Species	#1	#2	#3	#4	#5	#6	#7
Trichophyton tonsurans	±/2+	±/2+	4+	4+			
Trichophyton verrucosum	±	±	4+	2+			
Trichophyton megninii						±	4+
Trichophyton equinum	0				4+		

Usage

Media recommended for the differentiation of certain species of the genus *Trichophyton*.

   * *Difco Laboratories, Detroit, MI.*

2% Water agar

Composition

Agar   20 g
Tap water   1000 ml

Preparation

a) Mix the ingredients and bring to a boil to dissolve completely.
b) Sterilize at 121°C for 15 minutes.

Quality control

a) Appearance: colorless, transparent solid medium
b) Performance: no evaluation necessary before usage.

Usage

Elicits sporulation in certain saprobic fungi.

Bibliography

McGinnis, 1980
Vanbreuseghem, 1978

286

Calcofluor white 0.1%

Composition

Calcofluor white	0.1 g
Deionized water	100 ml

Preparation

Dissolve the calcofluor white in the water.

Quality control

a) Appearance: colorless liquid

b) Performance:

Candida albicans   apple green fluorescence when observed under fluorescence microscope

Storage

Store in a brown bottle at room temperature for not more than one year.

Usage

Fluorescent dye used for direct detection of fungi in biological specimens. Can also be used for visualization of certain structures difficult to see in conventional light microscopy.

Bibliography

Hageage, Harrington, 1984
Harrington, Hageage, 1991
Salkin, 1988

Lactophenol cotton blue

Composition

Phenol, concentrated	20.0 ml
Lactic acid	20.0 ml
Glycerol	40.0 ml
Cotton blue (aniline blue)	0.05 g
Distilled water	20.0 ml

Preparation

a) Dissolve the phenol in the mixture of lactic acid, glycerol and water.

b) Add the aniline blue and mix well.

Quality control

Appearance: deep blue liquid, slightly viscous

Usage

A mounting medium for microscopic examination. Caution: avoid exposure to phenol vapors during use.

Bibliography

McGinnis, 1980

Glossary

Acropetal

Said of a chain of conidia where the youngest conidium is found at the tip of the chain.

Adelophialide

A conidiogenous cell functioning as a phialide, and often resembling a typical phialide, but differing by not being septate at the base.

Adiaspore

Thick walled conidium which expands significantly in diameter when incubated at elevated temperature (37-42°C).

Aleurioconidium

Conidium liberated after release of a supporting cell; it is usually recognized by its truncate base bearing an annular frill.

Alternate

Used to describe arthroconidia alternating with vegetative cells (disjunctors, separating cells); these degenerate and break, liberating the arthroconidia.

Anamorph

Asexual or "imperfect" reproductive state of a fungus.

Annellide

A conidiogenous cell more or less differentiated from hyphae and producing conidia basipetally. The apex of the annellide shows percurrent proliferation, that is, it elongates slightly with the production of each new conidium and is ringed with a succession of circular scars, each one left behind by the secession of a conidium. These rings are not always discernible under the optical microscope.

Annelloconidium

Conidium formed by an annellide.

Annular Frill

A small, circular membrane attached at the base or at the extremities of a free conidium (aleurioconidium, alternate arthroconidium); this structure is a vestige of a separating cell, that is, a cell which supported the conidium in early growth

	but later ruptured in the process of freeing the conidium.
Anthropophilic	Used to describe a fungus (dermatophyte) which grows preferentially or exclusively on human hosts rather than on animal hosts or on decomposing materials in the soil.
Apex	Tip.
Apophysis	Funnel-shaped inflated area at the apex of a sporangiophore, just beneath the sporangium.
Arthroconidium	Conidium arising from the disarticulation of the cells of a hypha and liberated by a process of fission (simple arthroconidia) or by the lysis and fracture of separating cells (alternate arthroconidia).
Ascocarp	Fruiting structure which, in the species seen in the clinical laboratory, forms asci internally. Such structures constitute the characteristic sexual reproductive forms of certain members of the division Ascomycota. The newer term "ascoma" is increasingly often used and may eventually replace "ascocarp." Cleistothecia and perithecia are types of ascocarps.
Ascospore	Sexual spore formed within an ascus in fungi of the division Ascomycota. There are usually 4 or 8 ascospores per ascus (sometimes 2 or multiples of 4).
Ascus	Cell in the shape of a sac (round, club-shaped or cylindrical) within which ascospores are produced.
Ballistospore	A spore detached by one of a variety of types of ejection mechanisms and shot off at a distance from the colony.
Basidiospore	A sexual spore formed on the upper surface of a basidium in fungi of the division Basidiomycota. There are usually 4 basidiospores, sometimes 2, and rarely multiples of 4.

Basidium	A club shaped cell upon which basidiospores form.
Basipetal	Used to describe a chain of conidia in which the youngest conidium is found at the base.
Biseriate	In *Aspergillus*, used to describe an arrangement where phialides are supported by metulae attached to the surface of the vesicles.
Blastic	Used to describe a mode of conidium formation fundamentally based on a budding process. The septum which delimits a blastoconidium appears only after the formation of the conidium is complete. Thus, only a portion of the mother cell becomes transformed into a conidium. (See: blastoconidium, annelloconidium, phialoconidium, poroconidium, thallic)
Blastoconidium	Conidium produced by a budding process; in yeasts, a bud.
Blastomycosis	Disease caused by *Blastomyces dermatitidis*. The infection is usually acquired by inhalation of conidia and manifests initially in the lungs as a pneumonia-like disease. Later, it may disseminate, often to the skin, the bones, or the brain.
Chlamydospore	A vegetative resistant form, often seen as an inflated, rounded, thick-walled cell, intercalated within hyphae or situated terminally. Technically not a true spore or conidium, but rather, a resting structure or sessile perennation propagule.
Chromoblastomycosis	A chronic infection of subcutaneous tissues caused by a small group of dematiaceous fungi of which *Fonsecaea pedrosoi, Phialophora verrucosa* and *Cladosporium carrionii* are the most common representatives. The infection, characterized by verrucous skin lesions, and by the formation of brown, sclerotic fission cells in tissue, is often limited to a single limb. The disease follows inoculation of the causative fungus under the skin by a traumatic event such as piercing by a thorn.

291

Clamp Connection	A structure situated along the side of a hypha at the point where two cells meet, forming a looping bridge connecting the sides of the two cells. The presence of such structures in the vegetative hyphae of a colony indicates that the colony belongs to a member of the division Basidiomycota.
Clavate	Club-shaped.
Cleistothecium	The sexual fruiting body of certain fungi of the division Ascomycota. Typical cleistothecia are more or less rounded structures producing asci in their interiors. Unlike perithecia, they lack a defined opening for spore liberation and must be broken open before their ascospores are released.
Coccidioidomycosis	Disease caused by *Coccidioides immitis*. The infection is usually acquired by inhalation of arthroconidia of the fungus. Initially pulmonary, it often resolves spontaneously but in more serious cases disseminates to other parts of the body, including the skin, the bones, the joints, the liver, and the central nervous and genito-urinary systems.
Coenocytic	Not or sparsely septate, used to describe hyphae of Mucorales and similar structures where the cytoplasm of an organism is not generally segregated into individual cells.
Collarette	A cell wall remnant attached around the tip of a phialide. The collarette may resemble a vase or a tube, but is not always visible under the light microscope.
Columella	The inflated apex of a sporangiophore, forming a protuberance within the interior of a sporangium and physically supporting its weight.
Conidiogenous	Used to describe a specialized cell producing conidia. For example, annellides and phialides are conidiogenous cells.

Conidiophore	A specialized hypha upon which the conidia develop. The term may refer to a conidiogenous cell or to a specialized structure supporting a conidiogenous cell or cells.
Conidium	A unicellular or multicellular fungal element specialized to detach from the mycelium and disseminate, thus serving as an asexual reproductive structure.
Coremium	A fascicle of hyphae bound together in an upright sheaf and producing conidia at the apex. The word "synnema" is a common synonym.
Cycloheximide	A broad-spectrum anti-eukaryotic metabolic toxin produced by *Streptomyces griseus* and principally used as a selective agent for the isolation of dermatophytes (cf. Mycosel agar). Also known by the trade name Actidione.
Dehiscence	The tearing-away process that occurs when mature conidia separate and are liberated. This general term also applies to other structures separating by means of a circular tearing action.
Dematiaceous	Used to describe a fungus producing an olive-grey, brown or black pigment (melanin) in the cell wall of its hyphae or conidia. Sometimes colonies of dematiaceous fungi are pale at first, becoming darker as they age. The word derives from the anamorph-family Dematiaceae, an artificial taxon erected to contain all such dark fungi producing conidia on open branches, not in enclosed pycnidia. Therefore, fungi reproducing asexually only by means of pycnidia are never called dematiaceous, even when dark coloured. The same is true of fungi with only sexual reproduction.
Denticle	A small tooth-like outgrowth supporting a conidium.
Dermatomycosis	Infection of the skin, hair or nails by a fungus.

Dermatophyte	Fungus belonging to the genera *Epidermophyton*, *Microsporum* or *Trichophyton* infecting the skin or other keratinous elements of the integument of a living organism, e.g., nails, hair, feathers, claws.
Dermatophytosis	Infection of the skin, hair or nails by a dermatophyte.
Determinate	Used to describe a conidiophore or a conidiogenous cell which permanently ceases to grow before or just after the formation of the first conidium.
Dimorphic	Possessing two forms. Currently used in medical mycology to describe fungi which are thermally dimorphic, that is, which grow in a filamentous form at 25°C and in a particulate form (budding yeast, fission yeast or spherule) at 37°C on special media or in vivo. In general mycology, the word refers to any fungus able to convert between filamentous and particulate vegetative forms at any temperature.
Disjunctor	An empty cell which fragments or lyses, thereby liberating a conidium (arthroconidium or aleurioconidium).
Distoseptate	Used to describe a multicellular conidium which has cells not separated by conventional septa, but rather contained within sacs which have walls distinct from the outer wall of the conidium.
Echinulate	With small, more or less pointed, spine-like ornamentations on the surface.
Ellipsoidal	Used to describe a three-dimensional object which, if drawn in two dimensions, appears as an ellipse.
Endospore	Usually refers to spores formed within spherules of *Coccidioides immitis* and released at maturity.
Evanescent	Disappearing rapidly, fugacious. Often used to describe asci which rupture soon after their formation.
Exudate	Droplets of liquid formed on the surface of colonies.

Favic Chandelier	A hypha terminating in a branching structure resembling a chandelier or antlers. A typical feature of colonies of *Trichophyton schoenleinii*.
Fusoid	In the shape of a spindle; similar to an ellipsoid, but with two tapered and more or less pointed ends.
Geniculate	Used to describe a conidiophore which is sharply bent at one or more places (the word literally means, "as if with little knee joints"). This type of conidiophore typically results from sympodial development.
Geophilic	Used to describe a fungus (a dermatophyte or a non-pathogenic *Trichophyton, Microsporum* or *Epidermophyton*) which develops primarily or exclusively on substrates in the soil rather than on animals or humans.
Germ Slit	A specialized, narrow, thin-walled groove formed in the wall of a conidium or ascospore and splitting open to allow the emergence of a hypha. A commonly seen version of this structure is the equatorial germ slit, which runs right around the outer margin or equator of a lens-shaped or oblate (almost globe-shaped, slightly flattened) conidium.
Glabrous	Smooth; lacking hairs.
Heterothallic	Used to describe a fungus for which sexual reproduction is possible only after the mating of cells from two sexually compatible strains.
Hilum	A conspicuous, protuberant scar remaining on the base of a conidium at the point where it separated from the conidiogenous cell.
Histoplasmosis	A disease caused by *Histoplasma capsulatum*. The infection, usually acquired by the inhalation of conidia of the fungus, most often remains benign or asymptomatic. In certain patients, it may progress to a chronic or acute form, and may disseminate to the reticulo-endothelial system, the spleen, the liver, the adrenal glands, the gastrointestinal tract, the mucous membranes, and the bone marrow.

Homothallic	Used to describe a fungus in which a single isolate can spontaneously undergo sexual reproduction.
Hülle Cell	A refractile, thick-walled cell, variable in form, observed in certain species of *Aspergillus*.
Hyaline	Unpigmented, colorless. Often used to describe structures appearing colorless under the microscope.
Hyalohyphomycosis	A heterogenous group of infections caused by fungi lacking melanin (dark) wall pigmentation and characterized by the presence in tissue of septate, branching and/or toruloid hyphae. In practice, this term is applied to unusual mycoses and does not replace common, established terms such as aspergillosis. It does eliminate superfluous terms such as fusariosis and paecilomycosis, which are correctly rendered as "hyalohyphomycosis caused by *Fusarium*" and "... by *Paecilomyces*", respectively.
Hypha	Septate or aseptate filament of a fungus.
Imperfect	Used to describe the asexual state or anamorph of a fungus.
Indeterminate	Used to describe a conidiophore or a conidiogenous cell the growth of which is not interrupted when the first conidium is formed.
Macroconidium	The larger of two types of conidium produced by the same fungus. Often multicellular.
Merosporangium	Cylindrical sporangium containing spores in a linear series.
Metula	A conidiophore segment from which are produced the phialides in biseriate Aspergilli and pluriverticillate Penicillia.
Microconidium	The smaller of two types of conidium produced by the same fungus. Often unicellular.
Mold	A microscopic fungus principally producing filaments.

Mucorales
An order within the class Zygomycetes which includes the genera *Absidia, Cunninghamella, Mucor, Rhizopus,* and *Rhizomucor.* These fungi are distinctive in their rapidly growing colonies composed of large aseptate or rarely septate hyphae, and sporangia.

Muriform
Septate both transversely and longitudinally.

Mycelium
The totality of hyphae in a fungal colony; also, a mass noun referring to an indefinite quantity of fungal hyphae.

Mycetoma
A chronic infection of soft tissue or bone, usually limited to a single limb and characterized by the formation of swollen, indurated lesions with draining sinuses issuing white or black grains.

Nailhead Hypha
A hyphae which is thickened and flattened at the tip, typically encountered in certain dermatophytes such as *Trichophyton schoenleinii.*

Nodular Organ
A specialized feature of the submerged mycelium of certain dermatophytes, formed of a compact knot of swollen, usually colored hyphae.

Obclavate
Formed in the shape of an inverted club, that is, with the swollen part at the base.

Oblong
Of elongate form.

Obovoid
Formed in the shape of an egg, but with the narrow part at the base.

Onychomycosis
Infection of the nails caused by a fungus.

Ostiole
An opening formed in the wall of a perithecium or a pycnidium, through which spores or conidia escape.

Ovoid
Formed in the shape of an egg, with the broad end at the base.

Paracoccidioidomycosis
A chronic infection of the respiratory system caused by *Paracoccidioides brasiliensis.* It is char-

acterized by a primary infection of the lungs, accompanied by secondary lesions in the buccal, nasal or gastrointestinal mucosa.

Parasite An deleterious organism in intimate contact with another living organism and living entirely at its expense.

Pectinate Comb-like in shape. Principally used to describe specialized hyphae of certain dermatophytes.

Pedicellate Used to describe a conidium supported by a short filament.

Percurrent Used to describe a mode of conidiogenous cell development in which the cell forms a small extension through its own apex. In an annellide, this process occurs in conjunction with the formation of each new conidium.

Perfect Used to describe the sexual state or teleomorph of a fungus.

Perithecium Fruiting body formed by certain fungi of the division Ascomycota. Usually a flask-shaped or rounded structure, forming asci within its interior. Unlike a cleistothecium, the perithecium liberates its ascospores through a defined opening, referred to as an ostiole.

Phaeohyphomycosis A heterogenous group of infections characterized by brown hyphae, pseudohyphae or yeasts within host tissues. This name is usually used for relatively uncommon or rare mycoses for which no other recognized name exists.

Phialide An often bottle shaped conidiogenous cell, producing conidia basipetally. The length of the cell remains fixed during the entire time in which conidia are produced. A collarette is sometimes visible at the apex.

Phialoconidium A conidium produced by a phialide.

Pleomorphism	An apparently mutational phenomenon arising in dermatophytes in the laboratory, characterized by the disappearance of characteristic identification elements such as the colony pigmentation and conidial production.
Poroconidium	Conidia formed through a small pore in the conidiogenous cell.
Pseudohypha	A series of elongate blastoconidia remaining attached to one another, giving the appearance of a beaded hypha.
Pycnidium	In the Sphaeropsidales, a rounded structure, often flask-shaped, possessing an opening (ostiole) at its apex and forming conidia in its interior. A pycnidium resembles a perithecium but does not derive from a sexual process.
Pyriform	Pear shaped.
Racquet Hypha	A hypha composed of cells inflated at one end, giving the impression of a linear series of snowshoes or tennis racquets.
Reflexive Branching	Branches from the sides of a hypha growing in opposite directions, some towards the apex (axial branching) and some away from the apex (abaxial branching), with an appearance suggestive of barbed wire.
Rhizoid	Hyphae with a root-like appearance.
Saprobe	An organism obtaining its nourishment from decaying organic matter. Also referred to as a "saprophyte", a term which in its strict sense refers only to plants.
Sclerotic Fission Cell	A type of cell with dark, thick walls, dividing by bilateral fission, found in tissue in cases of chromoblastomycosis.
Sclerotium	A hard mass of hyphae which are closely interwoven and cemented together. This structure is a resistant body which, in the species seen in clini-

cal laboratories, gives rise to new hyphae on the return of favorable growth conditions.

Septum
A cross-wall within a hypha, a conidiophore, a conidium, or a spore.

Seta
A rigid hair, usually more or less long and stiffly erect, or undulate or spiralling, present on the ascocarps or pycnidia of certain fungi seen in the clinical laboratory. Usually formed in abundance.

Shield Shaped Cell
Conidium in the form of a V, a shield, or a buckler, seen in the genus *Cladosporium* at points where a conidial chain branches to form two chains.

Simple
Unbranched; used where appropriate to describe conidiophores.

Spherule
A spherical structure with a thick wall produced by *Coccidioides immitis* within host tissues and under special conditions in vitro. At maturity, it contains endospores.

Spiral Hypha
A hypha curved into a spiral, whether flattened or in a corkscrew-like helix. This specialized structure, seen in some dermatophytes, is more rigid than ordinary hyphal coils seen in many fungi, and is terminal rather than intercalary.

Sporangiole
A small sporangium containing only a small number of sporangiospores and sometimes only a single sporangiospore.

Sporangiophore
A specialized hypha giving rise to a sporangium.

Sporangiospore
An asexual spore produced by cytoplasmic cleavage within a sporangium.

Sporangium
A sac-like structure containing asexual spores formed by a process of cytoplasmic cleavage.

Spore
A fungal propagative element, produced either as part of a sexual process (ascospore, basidiospore, zygospore), or by an asexual reproductive process

involving a process of cytoplasmic cleavage (sporangiospore).

Sporodochium
A tight, broad cluster of hyphae giving rise to a cushion-like aggregation of conidiogenous cells and dry or slimy conidia.

Sporotrichosis
A subcutaneous infection caused by *Sporothrix schenckii* and characterized by the appearance of conspicuously swollen lymph nodes, beginning near the point of inoculation. Disseminated or pulmonary forms of the disease are rare.

Sterigma
A projection formed on the surface of a basidium and giving rise to a basidiospore at its apex. The term is also occasionally applied to phialides and metulae of *Aspergillus* in older literature.

Sterile
Used to describe a fungal culture which produces no spores or conidia.

Stolon
A horizontal, aerial hypha which gives rise to rhizoids and sporangiophores.

Sympodial
A general term for a filament made up of a nearly linear series of branches, each growing from just beneath the tip of the previous one. This term is most commonly used in clinical mycology to describe a conidiophore which develops by forming a conidium at its apex, then initiating a new growing point just beneath the apex, and pushing the conidium to one side as it elongates. This process is then repeated several times. Often the conidiophore takes on a geniculate or zigzag appearance.

Teleomorph
The sexual reproductive state of a fungus, also called the "perfect" state.

Thallic
Used to describe a mode of conidial formation which arises via the transformation of a segment of hypha already delimited by one or more cross walls. The mother cell is completely transformed into a conidium. (See aleurioconidium, arthroconidium, chlamydospore, blastic.)

Thallus   Colony; the totality of the vegetative and repro-
                 ductive structures of a fungal individual.

Toruloid   Used to describe a hypha or a conidiophore char-
                 acterized by a series of successive swellings and
                 constrictions.

Truncate   Used to describe a cell whose base ends abruptly,
                 as if it had been cut off.

Uniseriate   In *Aspergillus*, used to describe phialides formed
                 directly on the vesicle in the absence of interven-
                 ing metulae.

Verticil   Often used to describe a group of conidiogenous
                 cells with their bases attached in a circle around a
                 conidiophore, giving the appearance of the
                 spokes of a wheel (example, *Verticillium*).

Vesicle   A structure in the form of a small, swollen sac.
                 The term is often used to describe the inflated
                 apex of a conidiophore (e.g., in *Aspergillus*) or of
                 a sporangiophore (e.g., in *Syncephalastrum*).

Villose   Bearing soft hairs. Hairy, shaggy. A general term
                 used here to describe the surfaces of certain spo-
                 rangioles produced by *Conidiobolus coronatus*.

Zoophilic   Used to describe a fungus (dermatophyte) which
                 develops preferentially on animals rather than on
                 humans or in the soil.

Zygomycosis A category of diseases caused by fungi of the class
                 Zygomycetes. Infections caused by zygomycetous
                 fungi in the order Mucorales (*Absidia, Cunning-
                 hamella, Mucor, Rhizomucor, Rhizopus*) are typi-
                 cally diagnosed in the debilitated patient
                 suffering from diabetic ketoacidosis, malnutri-
                 tion, serious burns, or conditions affecting the
                 immune system. They are acute, often fatal, and
                 characterized by necrosis of tissue and infarcts in
                 the brain, the lungs, and the intestines. By con-
                 trast, infections caused by zygomycetous fungi in
                 the order Entomophthorales (*Basidiobolus, Coni-
                 diobolus*) are usually chronic and principally affect

302

the mucous membranes and the subcutaneous tissues.

Zygospore A sexual spore formed from the fusion of two similar cells called gametangia; this spore is characteristic of fungi in the division Zygomycota.

Bibliography

Arx, J.A. von. 1981. On *Monilia sitophila* and some families of Ascomycetes. Sidowya 34:13-29.

Atlas, R.M. 1993. Handbook of microbiological media. CRC Press. Boca Raton, Fa.

Barron, G.L. 1968. The genera of hyphomycetes from soil. Williams and Wilkins, Baltimore, MD.

Bièvre, C. de. 1991. Les *Alternaria* pathogènes pour l'homme: mycologie épidémiologique. Journal de mycologie médicale 1:50-58.

Bocobo, F.C., R.W. Benham. 1949. Pigment production in the differentiation of *Trichophyton mentagrophytes* and *Trichophyton rubrum*. Mycologia 41:291-302.

Carmichael, J.W. 1982. *Chrysosporium* and some other aleuriosporic hyphomycetes. Canadian Journal of Botany 40:1137-1173.

Centers for Disease Control and Prevention, and National Institutes of Health. 1993. Biosafety in microbiological and biomedical laboratories. 3rd ed. U.S. Department of Health and Human Services, Washington, D.C.

Cole, G.T., R.A. Samson. 1983. Conidium and sporangiospore formation in the pathogenic fungi. pp.437-524 In D.H. Howard (ed.), Fungi pathogenic for humans and animals. Marcel Dekker, New York.

Dixon, D.M., A. Polak-Wyss. 1990. The medically important dematiaceous fungi and their identification. Mycoses 34:1-18.

Dixon, D.M., I.F. Salkin, R.A. Duncan, N.J. Hurd, J.H. Haines, M.E. Kemna, F.B. Coles. 1991. Isolation and characterization of *Sporothrix schenckii* from clinical and environmental sources associated with the largest U.S. epidemic of sporotrichosis. Journal of Clinical Microbiology 29:1106-1113.

Domsch, K.H., W. Gams, T.-H. Anderson. 1980. Compendium of soil fungi. Academic Press, London.

Drouhet, E. 1993. Penicilliosis due to *Penicillium marneffei*: a new emerging systemic mycosis in AIDS patients travelling or living in Southeast Asia. Review of 44 cases reported in HIV infected patients during the last 5 years compared to 44 cases in HIV negative patients reported over 20 years. Journal de mycologie médicale 4:195-224.

Ellis, M.B. 1971. Dematiaceous Hyphomycetes. Commonwealth Mycological Institute, Kew.

Ellis, M.B. 1976. More dematiaceous Hyphomycetes. Commonwealth Mycological Institute, Kew.

Gams, W. 1971. *Cephalosporium*-artige Schimmelpilze (hyphomycetes). G. Fischer, Stuttgart.

Gams, W., M.R. McGinnis. 1983. *Phialemonium*, a new anamorph genus intermediate between *Phialophora* and *Acremonium*. Mycologia 75:977-987.

Georg L.K., L.B. Camp. 1957. Routine nutritional tests for the identification of dermatophytes. Journal of Bacteriology 74:477-490.

Guarro, J., J. Gené. 1992. *Hormographiella*, a new genus of hyphomycetes from clinical sources. Mycotaxon 45:179-190.

Guarro, J., J. Gené. 1992. *Fusarium* infections. Criteria for the identification of responsible species. Mycoses 35:109-114.

Guého, E., G.S. de Hoog. 1991. Taxonomy of the medical species of *Pseudallescheria* and *Scedosporium*. Journal de mycologie médicale 1:3-9.

Hageage, G.J., B.J. Harrington. 1984. Use of calcofluor white in clinical mycology. Laboratory Medicine 15:109-112.

Hall, G.S., K. Pratt-Rippin, J.A. Washington. 1992. Evaluation of chemiluminescent probe assay for identification of *Histoplasma capsulatum* isolates. Journal of Clinical Microbiology 30:3003-3004.

Harrington, B.J., G.J. Hageage. 1991. Calcofluor white: tips for improving its use. Clinical Microbiology Newsletter 13:3-5.

Hennebert, G.L. 1973. *Botrytis* and *Botrytis*-like genera. Persoonia 7:183-204.

Hermanides-Nijhof, E.J. 1977. *Aureobasidium* and allied genera. Studies in Mycology 15:141-177.

Hoog, G.S. de, M.T. Smith, E. Guého. 1986. A revision of the genus *Geotrichum* and its teleomorphs. Studies in Mycology 29:1-131.

Hoog, G.S. de. 1983. On the potentially pathogenic dematiaceous Hyphomycetes. pp.149-216 In D.H. Howard (ed.), Fungi pathogenic for humans and animals. Marcel Dekker, New York.

Huppert, M., S.H. Sun, E.H. Rice. 1978. Specificity of exoantigens for identifying cultures of *Coccidioides immitis*. Journal of Clinical Microbiology 8:346-348.

Kane, J. 1984. Conversion of *Blastomyces dermatitidis* to the yeast form at 37°C and 26°C. Journal of Clinical Microbiology 20:594-596.

Kaufman, L., E. Reiss. 1986. Serodiagnosis of fungal diseases, p. 446-466, In N.R. Rose, H. Friedman and J.L. Fahey (ed.), Manual of Clinical Immunology, 3rd ed., American Society for Microbiology , Washington, D.C.

Khan, Z.U., H.S. Randhawa, T. Kowshik, S.N. Gaur, G.A. de Vries, 1988. The pathogenic potential of *Sporotrichum pruinosum* isolated from the human respiratory tract. Journal of Medical and Veterinary Mycology 26:145-151.

King, D.S. 1983. Entomophthorales. pp.61-72 In D.H. Howard (ed.), Fungi pathogenic for humans and animals. Marcel Dekker, New York.

Koneman, W.E., G.D. Roberts. 1985. Practical Laboratory Mycology. 3rd ed. Williams and Wilkins, Baltimore.

Kurung, J.M., D. Yegian. 1954. Medium for maintenance and conversion of *Histoplasma capsulatum* to yeast like phase. American Journal of Clinical Pathology 24:505-508.

Kwon-Chung, K.J., J.E. Bennett. 1992. Medical Mycology. Lea & Febiger, Philadelphia.

McGinnis, M.R. 1980. Laboratory handbook of medical mycology. Academic Press, New York.

McGinnis, M.R., D. Borelli, A.A. Padhye, L. Ajello. 1986. Reclassification of *Cladosporium bantianum* in the genus *Xylohypha*. Journal of Clinical Microbiology 23:1148-1151.

McGinnis, M.R., A.A. Padhye, L. Ajello. 1982. *Pseudallescheria* Negroni et Fischer, 1943, and its later synonym *Petriellidium* Malloch, 1970. Mycotaxon, 14:94-102.

McGinnis, M.R., M.G. Rinaldi, R.E. Winn. 1986. Emerging agents of phaeohyphomycosis: pathogenic species of *Bipolaris* and *Exserohilum*. Journal of Clinical Microbiology 24:250-259.

Medical Research Council of Canada and Laboratory Centre for Disease Control. 1990. Laboratory biosafety guidelines. Minister of supply and welfare, Ottawa, Canada.

Miller, J.M. 1991. Quality control of media, reagents, and stains. pp. 1203-1225. In A. Balows, W.J. Hausler Jr., K.L. Herrmann, H.D. Isenberg, H.J. Shadomy (ed.). Manual of Clinical Microbiology, 5th ed. American Society for Microbiology, Washington, D.C.

Moore, M.K. 1988. Morphological and physiological studies of isolates of *Hendersonula toruloidea* Nattrass cultured from human skin and nail samples. Journal of Medical and Veterinary Mycology 26:25-39.

Moser, S.A., F.L. Lyon, D.L. Greer. 1988. Systemic mycoses, pp.173-238. In B.B. Wentworth (ed.), Diagnostic procedures for mycotic and parasitic infections. American Public Health Association, Washington, D.C.

National Committee for Clinical Laboratory Standards (NCCLS). 1990. Quality assurance for commercially prepared microbiological culture media; Approved Standard: M22 - A. National Committee for Clinical Laboratory Standards, Villanova, PA.

Nelson P.E., T.A. Toussoun, W.F.O. Marasas. 1983. *Fusarium* species: an illustrated manual for identification. Pennsylvania State University Press, PA.

O'Donnell, K.L. 1979. Zygomycetes in culture. Palfrey Contributions to Botany No.2, University of Georgia, Athens.

Oorschot, C.A.N. van. 1980. A revision of *Chrysosporium* and allied genera. Studies in Mycology 20:1-89.

Padhye, A.A., W.B. Helwig, N.G. Warren, L. Ajello, F.W. Chandler, M.R. McGinnis. 1988. Subcutaneous phaeohyphomycosis caused by *Xylohypha emmonsii*. Journal of Clinical Microbiology 26:709-712.

Padhye, A.A., G. Smith, D. McLaughlin, P.G. Standard, L. Kaufman. 1992. Comparative evaluation of a chemiluminescent DNA probe and an exoantigen test for rapid identification of *Histoplasma capsulatum*. Journal of Clinical Microbiology 30:3108-3111.

Raper, K.B., D.I. Fennell. 1973. The genus *Aspergillus*. Krieger, New York.

Rebell, G., D. Taplin. 1970. Dermatophytes, their recognition and identification. 2nd ed. University of Miami Press, Miami, FA.

Rippon, J.W. 1988. Medical mycology: the pathogenic fungi and the pathogenic Actinomycetes. 3rd ed. W.B. Saunders, Philadelphia.

Samson, R.A. 1974. *Paecilomyces* and some allied hyphomycetes. Studies in Mycology 6:1-119.

Scholer, H.J., E. Müller, M.A.A. Schipper. 1983. Mucorales pp. 9-60. In D.H. Howard (ed.), Fungi pathogenic for humans and animals. Marcel Dekker, New York.

Segretain, G., E. Drouhet, F. Mariat. 1987. Diagnostic de laboratoire en mycologie médicale. Maloine, Paris.

Sequeira, H., J.Cabrita, C. de Vroey, C. Wuytack-Raes. 1991. Contribution to our knowledge of *Trichophyton megninii*. Journal of Medical and Veterinary Mycology 29:417-418

Sigler, L. 1989. Problems in application of the terms "blastic" and "thallic" to modes of conidiogenesis in some onygenalean fungi. Mycopathologia 106:155-161.

Sigler, L., J.W. Carmichael. 1976. Taxonomy of *Malbranchea* and some other hyphomycetes with arthroconidia. Mycotaxon 4:349-488.

Sigler, L., J.W. Carmichael. 1983. Redisposition of some fungi referred to *Oidium microspermum* and a review of *Arthrographis*. Mycotaxon 18:495-507.

Simione, F.P., E.M. Brown. 1991. ATCC Preservation methods: freezing and freeze-drying. 2nd ed. American Type Culture Collection, Maryland.

Smith, D. 1991. Maintenance of filamentous fungi. pp. 134-159. In B.E. Kirsop, A. Doyle (ed.), Maintenance of microorganisms and cultured cells: a manual of laboratory methods, 2nd ed. Academic Press , London.

Stalpers, J.A. 1984. A revision of the genus *Sporotrichum*. Studies in Mycology 24:1-101.

Standard,P.G., L. Kaufman, S.D. Whaley. 1985. Exoantigen test: rapid identification of pathogenic mould isolates by immunodiffusion. U.S. Department of Health and Human Services, CDC, Atlanta.

Steadham, J.E., P.A. Geis, J.L. Simmank. 1986. Use of carbohydrate and nitrate assimilations in the identification of dematiaceous fungi. Diagnostic Microbiology and Infectious Disease 5:71-75.

Stockman, L., K.A. Clark, J.M. Hunt, G.D. Roberts. 1993. Evaluation of commercially available acridinium ester-labeled chemiluminescent DNA probes for culture identification of *Blastomyces dermatitidis*, *Coccidioides immitis*, *Cryptococcus neoformans*, and *Histoplasma capsulatum*. Journal of Clinical Microbiology 31:845-850.

Summerbell, R.C., S.A. Rosenthal and J. Kane. 1988. Rapid method for differentiation of *Trichophyton rubrum*, *Trichophyton mentagrophytes*, and related dermatophyte species. Journal of Clinical Microbiology 26:2279-2282.

Sutton, B.C, B.J. Dyko. 1989. Revision of *Hendersonula*. Mycological Research, 93:466-488.

Vanbreuseghem, R. 1978. Guide pratique de mycologie médicale et vétérinaire. Masson, Paris.

Weitzman, I. 1984. The case for *Cunninghamella elegans, C. bertholletiae* and *C. echinulata* as separate species. Transactions of the British mycological Society, 83:527-528.

Weitzman, I., J. Kane. 1991. Dermatophytes and agents of superficial mycoses, pp.601-616, In A. Balows, W.J. Hausler jr., K.L. Herrmann, H.D. Isenberg, H.J. Shadomy. Manual of Clinical Microbiology, 5th ed. American Society for Microbiology, Washington, D.C.

Weitzman, I., S. Rosenthal. 1984. Studies in the differentiation between *Microsporum ferrugineum* Ota and *Trichophyton soudanense* Joyeux. Mycopathologia 84:95-101.

World Health Organization. 1993. Laboratory biosafety manual. 2nd ed. WHO, Geneva.

INDEX

Page numbers in **boldface** refer to a main discussion of the entry; page numbers with a t refer to a table.

312

313